HOME FOR
HEALTH

Creating a sanctuary for healing

Hilton Tudhope

Published by Build for Health Press, Dallas, TX.
hilton@buildforhealth.com   **www.buildforhealth.com**

First Edition. Printed in the United States of America.

Library of Congress Cataloguing-in-Publication Data applied for.

ISBN: 978-0-692-11151-2

The information in this book is accurate to the best of our knowledge. This book is intended only as an informative guide for those wishing to know more about our experience of building a healthy home. Nothing contained herein should be construed as a medical diagnosis or treatment. If readers believe they are being adversely affected by their living or working environments, they should consult a qualified healthcare professional. All materials used in construction should be researched and tested for individual sensitivities, the goals of the project and the context in which they will be used.

For Barbara. And for all those who suffer from hyper-sensitivity to their living environment.

Your struggle is real.

Contents

*"Domestic well-being is too important to be
left to experts; it is, as it always has been, the
business of the family and the individual."*

— **Witold Rybczynski**

Preface

You might question why someone with no real-world expertise in architecture or construction might write a book of value about building a home. It's a reasonable question, so let me address it at the outset.

My wife and I had an overarching goal in commissioning what came to be branded as *+House:* to create an attractive contemporary residence that wouldn't make Barbara sick when we moved in. For her, the compromised immune and detoxification systems she had been dealt at birth were not sufficient to overcome the potentially debilitating impact of construction materials and processes. And while Barbara's health was improving, we had to make sure our new living environment would be as free as possible from chemical off-gassing and electromagnetic fields so there was no back-sliding on the hard-won gains she had made.

Over eighteen months of designing and building a prototype healthy home, we became experts, of a sort.

Experts in our own kind of health challenges and specific needs in a healthy living environment. In setting an intention and seeing it through to realization. Experts in asking questions of trades and suppliers that forced them to rethink their standard materials and application. And certainly experts in helping to manage the process of getting from concept to realization in the many-layered experience of building a home that would support Barbara's healing journey.

What we didn't become — and don't now claim to be — are experts in healthy house building processes or materials, nor in the complex sciences of house biology or environmental medicine. We did become expert *clients*: clients with a strong intention to healthy building, a considerable wealth of background information and, in the case of my wife, years of deep personal experience in the struggle to create a healthy life in a healthy body.

We believe a similar positive experience is possible for anyone who wants or needs to build healthy. This book is intended to add a practical, hands-on dimension to the many fine books already available on the need, materials and processes that form the foundation of healthy, sustainable construction and landscaping. Among those books, *Prescriptions for a Healthy House: A Practical Guide for Architects, Builders & Homeowners* (3rd Edition) stands out for its comprehensive, methodical approach to materials selection and building processes. It provided a daily touchstone for our architects and builder, and we required each trade to be familiar with the ideas, materials, and procedures the book outlined for their scope of work. "The Book," as we called *Prescriptions*, established the beginning point for most decisions we made, though not always the end point. As a set of practical guidelines based on actual experience, this book, in our view, is a companion to *Prescriptions* or any of the other books on green or healthy building listed in the Appendix.

Home for Health is structured as an amalgam of lessons gleaned from the combined experience of the clients, architects, contractor, trades, and suppliers who worked on the project. I have told our stories, and theirs, in the first person where I could because we want to highlight the actual experience of what healthy design, materials, and processes entail, and their impact on the actual people we hired to work with them.

If you're thinking about undertaking such a project, be warned that it is not always simple, straightforward, or intuitive. There will be extensive research. There will be constant questioning of the status quo. Your efforts probably won't end at the outside walls. But it is an immensely worthwhile and satisfying journey toward creating a home that sustains your life and protects your family's health.

I realize that our journey is not one that every reader will want or need to emulate. We built a prototype house, but not for altruistic reasons. There were no other viable options and we learned things along the way that made old ideas obsolete. It is a house that first and foremost had to respond to our own set of health issues and financial resources. Yet there are many insights we all learned, some of them wholly serendipitous, that may help remove a few of the obstacles along the path from design concept to built space. The purpose of this book is to share those lessons.

*"The connection between health and dwelling
is one of the most important that exists."*

Florence Nightingale

Introduction

In the late evening of September 9, 2007, two King Air twin-turbine crop dusters took off from Salinas Municipal Airport, just east of Monterey, California. Their payload was a mix of synthetic pheromone and allegedly inert chemicals known as Checkmate OLR-F, which was intended to disrupt the reproductive cycle of the light brown apple moth that officials suspected was beginning to invade the area. The crop dusters' mission: spray the pesticide over sixty square miles of heavily populated urban areas and farmland along California's scenic Central Coast. Working into the early hours of the morning on three separate nights from an altitude of 500 feet, the planes saturated the coastal towns of Marina, Seaside, Pacific Grove, and parts of Pebble Beach with the mysterious, unproven chemical.

We understood the importance of agriculture to the state's economy. But this was California. Of all states in the nation, it had a reputation for being the most protective of the environment. Any program of this magnitude, having the potential to affect millions of people, would surely be properly vetted for its environmental and human impacts, right? Not so. The California Department of Food and Agriculture, with funding from the United States Department of Agriculture, designated the moth offensive an "emergency." That exempted the state from conducting an environmental impact assessment as required under its own Environmental Quality Act. And even though Checkmate was not yet registered as a pesticide, neither the federal Environmental Protection Agency nor the California Department of Pesticide Regulation required it to be tested for its effects on human or animal health.

By the time a combination of court order and public outrage halted the spraying the following spring, there were over 640 documented health complaints, ranging from asthma attacks to severe headaches and from eye irritation to 'brain fog.' My wife, Barbara, deposed under oath, was among those who detailed her health reactions to the spraying. At the time, she ran a successful yoga studio in Pacific Grove, which she had opened two years earlier. Though she spent most of her time in Pacific Grove teaching indoors, she was in the town frequently enough to be exposed to the residue of the Checkmate spray.

It couldn't have come at a more challenging time in her quest to get healthy. Barbara was in the lengthy process of rebuilding the strength of her immune and digestive systems under the care of a board-certified physician at the Environmental Health Center in Dallas. A genetic profile a few years earlier revealed that Barbara's body did not possess all the "tools" needed to process and eliminate environmental toxins. More concerning still was the potential impact on her kidneys — a primary detoxification route — which were compromised by the effects of an autoimmune disease identified some twenty years earlier. Any significant increase in the chemical load her body had to process spelled danger.

When Barbara detailed her symptoms after the spraying — shortness of breath, bad headaches, asthma-like symptoms, an inability to focus — Barbara's doctor at the Health Center told her emphatically that she was to leave the area and stay away for at least thirty days every time it was sprayed.

When the crop dusters returned to Carmel in late October, we heeded the doctor's advice and spent the next month in Dallas. Shortly after, faced with the prospect of years of bi-monthly spraying, Barbara reluctantly sold the yoga studio, and we purchased a condominium in Dallas as our escape hatch from Paradise. It was a very difficult time, for Barbara especially, when many of the anchors of life — home, work, health — felt like they were crumbling away.

However troubling, the message from above did ultimately have a positive effect on our lives. It began a sequence of choreographed moves that led to the design and construction of our new home. It forced us to identify the qualities we wanted in our living environment, like clean air, abundant water, and local organic food, that would support Barbara's health and our long-term well-being. Our decision would take us away from the friends and home we loved in Carmel. But it would bring us back into our family folds in Texas and Ontario. And we would spend a lot less time running ourselves ragged on 'visiting vacations' that inevitably left us feeling exhausted.

There are certainly many spectacular places in North America with abundant fresh water and clean air. Places that are quiet and regenerative and unlikely to be tainted by agricultural chemicals. Dallas is not one of them. But we had three of Barbara's children and a large portion of her family in Texas, as well as her doctors at the Environmental Health Center. We had the condo near the vibrant Arts District of the city. It seemed the right decision.

Not unlike Dallas, our choice of a homesite in Mulmur Township, about an hour and a half northwest of Toronto, also revolved around family and social considerations. My mother lives in Toronto, along with my brothers and their families. We have many good friends in both the city and the country. It was a logical choice that saved us the challenge of reinventing our lives once again.

We began our search in Ontario in 2008 during our annual summer visit. We contacted a local real estate agent we were acquainted with who had grown up in the area and knew it intimately. She suggested a few drive-bys to get a gauge of our interests. After miles of rolling, dusty roads across several townships, nothing caught our attention. Pressed as always for time on these visits, we returned to Carmel.

My experience has always been that the manifestation of an idea gains momentum as you gather information to support it. We knew the area in which we wanted to live. We had gone looking. When we told our friends back in Carmel about our decision — a difficult conversation — we added an emotional charge to our plan. If we were willing to leave these wonderful people, we were really committed. In the broader context of events, it appeared that Barack Obama was about to be elected as the first

African-American president of the United States. We experienced a tangible feeling of change and hope washing over much of the country. We were caught up in it and it colored our world. I had even applied to become a naturalized U.S. citizen.

On Election Day, after a business meeting in Milwaukee, I flew to Toronto to meet again with our agent. Of the six properties I saw on that uncharacteristically warm day in early November, one met most of our conditions. Though the house failed miserably to impress on first inspection, the land was ideal: eleven acres, with a large swimming pond fed by springs and a year-round stream. Beautiful gardens, specimen trees, and views to a distant hillside. The site was located on a quiet country road on the Niagara Escarpment, which is a protected corridor, 450 miles long, from Niagara Falls to the Bruce Peninsula that is designated a UNESCO World Biosphere Reserve. But as we would discover when construction started, it was a very difficult building site, with a long east-west axis from the road bounded tightly by the pond to the south and a sharply rising hill to the north.

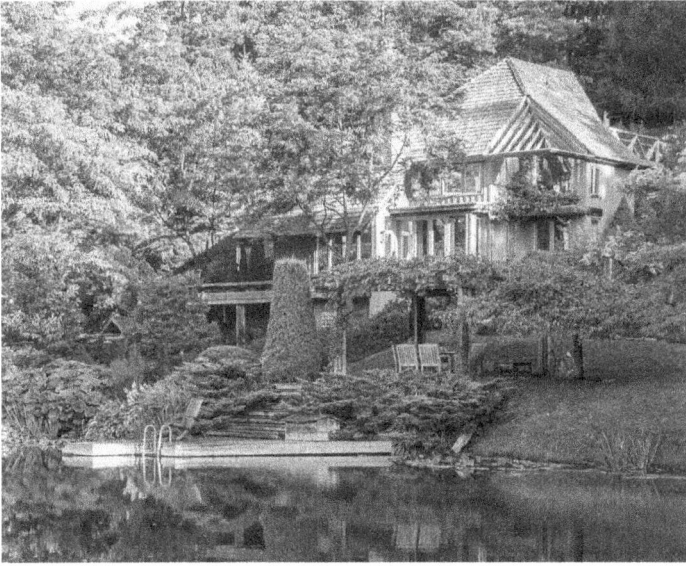

Lovely gardens, unsalvageable house.

For a property both beautiful and welcoming, the existing house challenged most every idea we held about even basic functional living. It was built on the north side of the pond, backing into a steep slope that rose some fifty feet from the water's edge to a mature forest above. Perhaps to minimize the hill retention or to maximize the opportunity for gardens, the architect had emphasized the verticality of the structure. There were strange architectural "gestures" everywhere, as one designer put it. The resulting house was, to our eyes, a hopeless warren of small, oddly-shaped spaces on four inconsistent levels, with capricious changes in floor and ceiling heights, and a nightmare of blatantly out-of-code, homemade renovations.

It was a tear-down. We resigned ourselves to a single summer there, moved in our furniture and got on with trying to create a sense of home, or at least some psychological bond to the land. That fall we engaged the architects and began a tremendously exciting process led by professionals we felt understood our intention to build a healthy house on a reasonable budget.

In June 2010, with the design finalized, the architects were about to go to the county offices to apply for building permits when Barbara became concerned about an email exchange concerning the use of petrochemical release agents on concrete form boards. A release agent is typically applied to the plywood forms used to contain freshly poured concrete while it sets; the agent prevents the concrete from adhering to the form board.

Barbara is smart, curious, and knowledgeable about her health issues, but her understanding of construction materials and processes was limited to the information in several books she had read on healthy building. But it was sufficient for her to realize that what had been proposed as a standard, unquestioned construction process was a potential threat to her health. Release agents like those that had been proposed are typically manufactured from petrochemicals that off-gas volatile organic compounds. The issue, from a healthy construction standpoint, is the likely contamination of the plywood forms from repeated use of the release agents.

Barbara ended her email reply to the contractor with, "I'm not sure who orders the materials for a project like this. I'm finding myself in a challenging position because I don't want to be overbearing. But I've also had the experience of not asking enough questions and suffering the consequences later." To their credit, our builder replied, "We are relying on you to make these points and ask these questions. Out of all of us, you know the most about healthy building. By the end of the project, we will all be experts."

That exchange came to define the relationship between ourselves as "advocate-owners" and the architects, contractor, trades, and suppliers who worked for us — naïve questions, tentative answers, more questions, new alternatives. Every material was scrutinized for its health impact, along with most every building process.

We call our new home *+House* because it is more than just a structure for dwelling. It is award-winning contemporary design. It is a prototype healthy home. And as we had hoped, it is a home that nourishes and refreshes us and, by all reports, everyone who visits. Wherever possible, we based the design and construction on sustainable building practices and the tenets of Leadership in Energy and Environmental Design (LEED), though that was not our primary objective. But by the end of the project, we were impressed by the broad intersection of "green" and "healthy" and surprised by the few instances where they failed to share the same goals.

Lewis Carroll's assertion that, "if you don't know where you're going, any road will take you there," is a fair one when it comes to home construction. It's a complex undertaking for the uninitiated, and few of us have the knowledge or desire to question the myriad materials and processes that go into our living environment. Fewer still invest the energy to investigate material safety data sheets or hunt down studies of the long-term health effects of exposures to chemical ingredients or electromagnetic fields. Yet these are exactly the activities that homeowners should be undertaking to protect themselves and their families.

In our case, the decision to build healthy was driven by need, as described more fully in Lesson 1: Know Yourself. The success of the project, however, was a product of intention. Initially, it was our own intention, shared with a few friends and family and hastened by the purchase of a property. But it quickly spread to the team of accomplices we gathered around ourselves to bring the house from concept into manifestation. The more strongly we held to our intention that a healthy house was not only necessary but possible — and possible on a specific budget — the more actively everyone involved got behind the idea, without compromise. Yes, they were professionally obligated to produce the outcome we wanted. But the many challenges of building a prototype house demand a deeper commitment that only comes from a shared vision.

Establishing such a shared commitment was essential because we weren't around to oversee most of the construction. +*House* is not our primary residence. Barbara and I live in Dallas for seven months of the year. With the exception of two very brief visits in February and May 2011, we didn't see the house in person for over eight months. We headed south with the foundation in place and returned to see the last of the cabinetry being installed. In the interim, we received a continual flow of emails and photographs that dealt with the many questions and showed us the progress of construction.

For some contractors, absentee owners would be a dream. But with every material and process under constant scrutiny for its health impact, it put a lot of responsibility on the builder. As our site supervisor said, "When Barbara showed up, we were scared as hell she'd run out of the house. We'd work for six months and not know."

We never doubted it would be great, but we didn't really know, either. What we did know was that we held a common goal of a great outcome.

As a result, we developed a strong bond of trust with our architects, builder and trades. We could count on them to work through challenges without simply defaulting to what was familiar. We could count on them to deal with our naive questions and our 'line in the sand' attitude for what constituted a healthy living environment. In contrast to many stories we hear about clients and contractors on contentious projects, our relationships with the team were never adversarial, nor were there issues between the other team members that were important enough to rise to our ears. Our common intention to do something different and groundbreaking held us together. It was the best lesson we learned, one that we will detail in the coming chapters.

Notes

1   The program was eventually defunded in California's 2012 budget but lived on in the courts. In late 2015, the Third District Court of Appeal ruled unanimously that CDFA's Programmatic Environmental Impact Report on the state's Light Brown Apple Moth Eradication/Control Program violated the California Environmental Quality Act, effectively killing the program.

Lesson 1:

Know Yourself

To anyone who has never suffered from an environmental illness like allergies, loves the smell of a new car, can't wait to walk on freshly glued carpet, and has a half-dozen favorite fragrances, the concept of building a healthy house probably seems very indulgent, if it even crosses their minds. Why bother when the construction industry and its suppliers have proven products and processes that can create a completely acceptable house at an affordable price?

The reason to be concerned is the total toxic load now found in our environment and our bodies' ability to deal with it. Toxic load or "body burden" is the total amount of current and accumulated toxic chemicals that we absorb from our environment. Manufacturers produce thousands of synthetic chemicals each year, many of them new and the great majority of which are without health or safety data or information on their interactions with other chemicals.

In his excellent book on the subject, *What's Gotten into Us: Staying Healthy in a Toxic World*, McKay Jenkins states: "By the mid-1970s, there were some 62,000 chemicals in use; today the number is thought to be closer to 80,000. The EPA [Environmental Protection Agency] has a full set of toxicity information for just seven percent of these chemicals, and the U.S. chemical industry... is so woefully under-regulated that 99 percent of chemicals in use today have never been tested for their effects on human health."[1] According to *The Washington Post*, under current law the EPA is ensnared in a classic "Catch-22" when it comes to evaluating the safety of these compounds: it can't subject chemicals to testing without evidence of potential risk, which is hard to obtain without testing. "Consequently," the *Post* editorial stated, "the EPA has managed to examine a mere 200 chemicals since 1976, though thousands are produced and sold every year."[2]

Even a partial list of chemical pollution from allegedly safe products in the average home today is overwhelming: flame retardants, stain repellents, formaldehyde and other volatile organic compounds, plastics, beverage containers and can linings, perfumes, shampoos and air fresheners, and all manner of standard cleaning products.[3]

Outside, pollutants like vehicle exhaust, products of coal

combustion, pesticides, herbicides, and insecticides add to the chemical load our bodies must process.

We breathe in this noxious stew of chemicals through our lungs, ingest it through our mouths, and even absorb it through our skin. If we're fortunate enough to have a strong immune system and all the genetic 'equipment' required for natural and efficient detoxification, we may process most of this burden through our liver and kidneys. If we're not so fortunate, these chemicals will tend to accumulate in our joints, bones, and fatty tissue. Some chemicals persist, meaning they don't break down readily for elimination. Others bioaccumulate, meaning they will gradually increase in concentration in our tissues. That can result in chronic toxicity that leads, in some cases, to debilitating health issues like asthma, chronic fatigue, cancers, autoimmune disorders, and multiple chemical sensitivity.[4]

The buildup of chemicals in our bodies is even more concerning in the case of young children and infants with developing physiological processes, especially those related to their immune and nervous systems. Compared to adults, children eat, drink, and breathe more air as a percentage of their body weight. They play on the carpet and crawl on the grass, absorbing chemical pollutants through their skin. According to Dr. Leonardo Trasande, an associate professor of pediatrics, environmental medicine, and health policy at New York University, as the chemical load has increased, "we've seen an increase in chronic childhood diseases: asthma, developmental disabilities, certain birth defects, certain childhood cancers."[5]

And this is to say nothing of the additive — and potentially debilitating — impacts on our bodies from electromagnetic fields in and around our homes, radio frequencies from cell phone use and smart meters, and microwave transmissions.

How prevalent might chemical sensitivity be? Dr. Lisa Lavine Nagy, a practicing medical doctor and founder of the Preventive and Environmental Health Alliance in Massachusetts, suggests that three to five percent of the U.S. population is disabled from chemical sensitivity, fifteen percent present some symptoms, and at least forty percent of Americans have at least mild symptoms of which they are unaware. Approximately 74 million people are thought to be affected.[6]

For those who aren't especially healthy to begin with, the long-term effects of exposure to environmental toxins can be overwhelming, both physically and psychologically. Diagnosis and treatment are challenging because few doctors are educated in the precepts of environmental medicine. Acute exposures to toxic chemicals may be easy to identify, but long-term exposure to low levels of a chemical, possibly combined with numerous other exposures in the home or workplace, leave most medical practitioners focusing on relieving the patient's symptoms rather than addressing the root causes of the complaint.

As Barbara sees it, "there are very few people who make the connection between a breakdown in their immune system and a chronic illness and toxicity in their body, other than doctors who have a background in environmental medicine. So, people adapt and learn to live with those chronic illnesses rather than being able to specifically identify that the problem is caused by things in their environment, whether it's the cleaning products or pesticides they're using at home, or what they're using in the garden. Or even whatever is in the air. So you just continue to live in an environment that's causing illness without realizing that's what is happening. And because so many people are trying to deal with the same thing, you just think it's normal. It's not."

So why build healthy? The answer is very obvious to us now. Given good information and a range of excellent alternatives, why wouldn't you create a home — or renovate one — with products and processes that support your health, or at least won't affect it adversely? Yet we have watched for years as otherwise thoughtful friends and relatives undertook major construction or renovation projects — all conventionally built — only to report weeks or months later that they have been prescribed an inhaler for asthma symptoms or are suffering from some form of chronic fatigue or skin irritation. Even then, few seem willing or knowledgeable enough to make the connection between their symptoms and the out-gassing of chemical compounds emanating from the paint in their bedrooms, the cabinets in the kitchen and the broadloom in the living room. Sadly, and for the most part unnecessarily, many formerly healthy individuals gradually find themselves succumbing to chronic ailments.

Through insight or necessity, people sometimes begin to ask questions, to look beyond the symptoms. In our case, Barbara's questioning began out of necessity. "I was fortunate," she said, "to work with two medical doctors with deep personal experience in environmental medicine, as both patients and practitioners. But I also had to do a lot of my own exploration on what it would take to get well. Until you start reading and learning, you have no idea how saturated our environment is with chemicals. You don't know until you know, then once you know, you have to change."

Let's be clear that this book is about helping ease the challenges of building a healthy home, as seen through the lens of our experience. It is not intended to be a comprehensive survey of the science and research behind the *need* to build a healthy living environment. There are many excellent books and informative websites listed in the bibliography that detail the health impacts of chemical toxicity in our air, water, food, and homes. Start there if you're in the early stages of your exploration.

If you suspect that you may already be dealing with the effects of exposure to toxins such as molds, volatile organic compounds, lead or radon, try answering these questions, which have been adapted from Dr. Nagy's environmental screening history:

- When did you last feel well?

- What changes occurred in your life after that time?

- What do you think has precipitated your condition? For example, have you renovated your home or office with new cabinets, carpet or paint? Do you spray pesticides indoors? Is there less ventilation or more chemicals in your workplace than there used to be?

- Are you sensitive to perfumes, diesel exhaust, detergents, newspapers, fabric softeners, and air fresheners?

- Do you feel better in the outside air? Are you worse inside during the winter?

- Do you feel exhausted in department stores, tire centers, or moldy buildings?

- Do you have a moldy basement, or does the house smell musty when you first come home?

- Have you been avoiding dealing with a water leak?

- Do electrical appliances and cell phones make you feel headachy or ill?

- Does your spouse think you're a hypochondriac or just plain wacky?

- Do you feel you are definitely ill but no doctor has been able to help you?

If you want to have a more informed discussion with your healthcare practitioner, we encourage you to answer these questions candidly. You may also want to fill out the Exposure History Form developed for doctors by the Agency for Toxic Substances & Disease Registry at the Centers for Disease Control in Atlanta.[7] You may be surprised by what you find.

Our Questioning Begins

While few people knew it from her appearance, with the turn in the millennium came a worsening turn in Barbara's health. Since the diagnosis of an autoimmune disease affecting her kidneys in her mid-thirties, she had lived a full and active life, raising four children and navigating a difficult divorce. The doctor's best advice for this latest challenge was to take a low dose of preventative antibiotics and to lead a stress-free life. Easy for him to suggest: he was too young to have to juggle kids and carpools.

A couple of years after we were married, Barbara's annual medical tests indicated that her kidney function was declining further. On the advice of a homeopathic doctor, she tested for the possibility that mercury vapor was leaking from the extensive silver amalgams that had been in her teeth for decades. The test was positive, and we decided that she should have the amalgams removed from her mouth to eliminate what we believed was the toxic effect of mercury on her kidneys. Despite careful extraction of the fillings, within a few months Barbara's digestive system went through what appeared to be another serious deterioration. She lost weight and vitality. The best suggestion medical practitioners had to calm down her system was a bland diet of fish and vegetables. It worked, more or less, for a while.

The problem with finding an effective treatment was that no individual doctor had a picture of Barbara that included the environmental perspective. As a result, we had no comprehensive approach to the complex set of symptoms she was presenting. In the fall of 2002, a family connection led Barbara to Dr. Katherine Henry, an internist in Dallas with a personal interest and professional credentials in environmental medicine. Barbara felt that her new M.D. evinced a strong commitment to understanding what lay beneath these symptoms, and so they began extensive testing to obtain the baseline functioning of her cardiovascular, digestive, immune, and detoxification systems.

Each of these tests shone some welcome light on the mysteries of Barbara's physical makeup. But none was more telling nor ultimately more influential in our decision to build a healthy house than the identification of the genomic profile of Barbara's detoxification system.

In my simplistic understanding of it, detoxification is the metabolic process our bodies use to act on and eliminate toxins, whether those toxins are from food and medicines we consume, natural waste our own bodies create during metabolism, or environmental stressors like air and water pollution, molds, pesticides and solvents. In Phase I detoxification, the liver is involved in breaking down toxins for elimination, and for some compounds that's all that is needed. But for others, the body requires a second phase that further transforms the chemical structure of a toxin by adding water-soluble molecules that promote elimination.

These genetic test results were particularly discouraging. Of the eight genetic 'tools' for Phase I detox, one of Barbara's was impaired — a "polymorphism" in the medical lexicon — increasing not only her susceptibility to toxins but also the likelihood those toxins would accumulate in her body. That put more stress on Phase II genes, which would have a heavier load to clear. Several of these second-phase genes were also compromised. Missing entirely was a gene involved with her body's ability to produce the antioxidant glutathione, which is essential to eliminating many environmental toxins.

All of this was a revelation. Along with the liver, intestines and skin, the kidneys are a major exit route for toxins. But rapid detoxification protocols like EDTA, a chelation therapy approved as a treatment for lead and heavy metal poisoning, would put too much stress on Barbara's kidneys. Dr. Henry started Barbara on a series of two-hour intravenous treatments using ingredients such as vitamin C, vitamin B and glutathione, all intended to support her body in its struggle to detoxify without compromising her kidney function. She prescribed a broad regimen of supplements, each of which would address specific detox priorities. Some months later, another test revealed Barbara to be gluten intolerant. This stressor, along with the deterioration of her intestinal flora from years of excessive (though prescribed) antibiotic use, finally explained some of her severe digestive issues. We felt like we were finally making some progress, even though the toxins being released into her bloodstream from the treatments inevitably led to headaches, brain fog, weakness, and lethargy.

With Barbara's youngest son off to college, we moved from North Texas to Monterey Peninsula on California's Central Coast in mid-2003 in the hope of better air and a more moderate climate. We were fortunate to find another internist affiliated with the American Academy of Environmental Medicine who was sensitive to Barbara's issues and who took great care to ensure her kidneys were protected. The intravenous drips continued and, gradually, our lives took on less stressful rhythms. Barbara completed her training as a Viniyoga teacher. She opened Wellsprings Yoga studio in Pacific Grove and worked tirelessly to make it a success, eventually receiving her certification as a Viniyoga therapist in 2006.

The need for a second opinion on a proposed procedure to evaluate her heart function took Barbara, ironically, back to the Environmental Health Center (EHCD) in Dallas. She wanted a perspective from its founder, Dr. William Rea, a thoracic and cardiovascular surgeon who is regarded as one of the world's leading practitioners of environmental medicine. The EHCD has pioneered the use of comprehensive diagnostic testing, and medical and natural therapies — some of them definitely controversial — to deal with health problems related to the environment. They treat all manner of sensitivities, including pollens, molds, dust, foods, chemicals, air, water, and electromagnetic radiation, often for those with profoundly challenging health circumstances. Many of their patients have run out of conventional solutions.

To the outside observer not afflicted by debilitating chronic health issues, the Center itself is not a warm and comfortable place to spend months or sometimes years in treatment. It is designed to be an "environmental control unit" that strictly minimizes the impact of indoor and outdoor pollution, and electromagnetic fields, on its patients. Porcelain walls and floors, hardwood chairs and benches, and noisy air cleaners comprise most of the décor. Few comforts are allowed: no scents (manufactured chemicals), no books or magazines (volatile organic compounds), and no cell phones (radio frequency radiation). The ambience suggests a hospital operating room. As Barbara put it, "I felt I wasn't *that* sick. I didn't want to be in that sterile environment. There was nothing soft in sight. The patients seemed odd, some very thin and others wearing masks and making determined efforts to avoid me."

Dr. Rea's opinion as a cardiologist was that the stress of the proposed cardiac test wasn't worth the small amount of additional information it might reveal. "He was more concerned about the various sensitivities I had developed," Barbara recalls, "and even thought he could help with the kidney disease. He did a test that revealed I had been exposed to a type of mold that is especially toxic to the kidneys. He believed that sauna treatments, combined with the IVs I was already doing, could flush the mycotoxin from my body. But I'd also have to do other treatments like allergy testing and nutritional counseling to make sure we would get the best outcome and protect my remaining kidney function. It was all overwhelming."

Barbara's path to health has been strewn with challenges. Allergy testing was not the usual scratch test. It was subcutaneous injection of an allergen, followed by further injections to determine baseline reactivity as measured by physical responses like local skin swelling and headache severity. There were hundreds of potential allergens and days of reactions that lengthened into months of stress. And there were years of self-administered injections of antigens to help condition Barbara's immune system so that it would not attack virtually everything she came in contact with or ingested.

Nor were saunas of the usual variety. Patients are required to take a handful of supplements to promote elimination of toxins and spend fifteen minutes on a treadmill to accelerate their heart rates. Then into the infrared sauna — thirty minutes at more than 150 degrees Fahrenheit — which inevitably led to more headaches and weariness as the toxins were flushed into Barbara's bloodstream for elimination.

Even to an "insider" like myself, who had the benefit of some explanation to inform my blind hopefulness that it would all work out for the best, Dr. Rea's treatment program seemed Draconian. It took a while to see some results in Barbara's health, perhaps eighteen months or more. They came haltingly, often punctuated by a step or two back after a few months of hard-won progress. I didn't understand the nature of the detoxification process or why the setbacks took place; she was incredibly disciplined despite how she felt. She explained the backsliding as, "When your body begins to unload toxins, it also begins to react to the chemicals in your environment. Everyday substances that you may not have realized contain chemicals, like fragrances — which you may not have even noticed before — become intolerable. They begin to cause reactions, like headaches, dizziness, congestion, and skin rashes. It's a process they call unmasking."

Until this point, Barbara's struggles had been largely personal, shared with only a few friends, family, and the annoyed agents at airport security checkpoints who had to hand-inspect her frozen antigen vials. Unmasking took us public. At the nadir of her journey, in December

2007, Barbara — who in the previous month had dealt with having to flee our home in California, the likely demise of her beloved yoga studio, and extensive allergy testing — announced, in tears, that the tests revealed she was now allergic to cotton and wool. Natural fibers were inextricably linked with our lives. Barbara had a closet full of cotton and wool clothes. We slept in organic cotton sheets and wool blankets. Towels? Underwear? It felt like the last and heaviest straw. Questions arose about a life worth living.

Our adaptation is a testament to Barbara's discipline and will to health. She gradually remade her wardrobe from alternative fabrics, mostly synthetics. To this day, we sleep in bamboo sheets over a hemp comforter that protects her from the cotton mattress cover. And everywhere we travel, the "green suitcase" is our constant companion, filled with bamboo sheets, polyester blankets and heavy-duty tin foil to cover mattresses that — to Barbara — occasionally reek of the headache-inducing chemical signature of fabric softener.

Thanks to the unmasking phenomena, manufactured fragrances remain an ongoing challenge for Barbara. In her own words:

At one time, fragrances were derived naturally, from flowers and herbs. Now it's primarily a specialty chemical business, and these artificial fragrances are everywhere, from bathrooms to malls, from cars to airplanes. They may be pleasant if you can tolerate them, but for the chemically sensitive person like me, they're debilitating.

You have to strategize to limit your exposure. We try to find seats at the end of a row in theaters, in case someone sits near us with a cloud of perfume hovering around them. I avoid fragrance and makeup departments, and hardware stores. If we're given a new rental car when we travel, we insist on an older one so the 'new car' smell has gassed off. We'll change rooms in a hotel if they use air freshener or clean with chemical products after we've requested otherwise. One manager at a high-end hotel balked when we wanted to move rooms, protesting that Febreze was a natural product. Because people are just unaware of the many chemicals around us every day, you have to educate a lot of people.

Sometimes it's just out of your control and you pay the price. We were flying home from Asia a couple of years ago and the plane didn't smell 'right' to me. Just after they shut the cabin door, a flight attendant got on the intercom to tell everyone how excited they were to be flying on the airline's brand new Boeing 777. It was thirteen hours of 'new-car-smell' hell.

Think what you will about the treatment program that Barbara undertook and however halting her progress — many family and friends were dismayed by both — the regimen of antigen shots, sauna treatments, and a strict rotation diet gradually brought her back to vitality with her kidney function intact. She 'graduated' herself from the Environmental Health Center in 2009 and stopped all antigen shots the following year. With her immune system calmed down, Barbara was able to tolerate a wider variety of foods and her weight slowly returned to normal.

The 'Toxins' We Don't See

To this point, I've focused mainly on environmental toxins from chemicals and products of combustion. They weren't our only concern in building *+House*. Reducing the potential health effects of electromagnetic and radio frequencies was also an important consideration. An experience we had suggests why.

Not long after our return to Dallas from California, Barbara and I discovered that occasional condo living was very different from full-time condo living. We wanted a modest house in a good, downtown neighborhood, and began our search. Now, trying to find a reasonably healthy home from real estate listings is neither educated nor intuitive. All we could do was specify the areas we liked and eliminate the obvious, like new construction or proximity to high-voltage electrical lines. We went through a couple of dozen candidates until we finally found what seemed to us the perfect townhouse at the right price — contemporary design, open spaces, and ideally situated. Our offer included two conditions: the usual inspection of the property for physical defects and an extended period of time to complete what we called an "environmental assessment." We paid a non-refundable $1,000 fee to the owner for the additional time.

We felt we needed the extra time to determine the source, or even the validity, of what Barbara described as a feeling of "spikiness" at certain places in the house that made her "jittery." Unless we could determine that the source was harmless — and we had doubts — we couldn't go ahead with the purchase. From Barbara's learning at the Environmental Health Center, we knew that that feeling could be come from spikes in electromagnetic radiation or radio frequencies. Perhaps some electrical wiring had faulty connections. Maybe the pole-mounted transformer at the back alley was out of spec. It could have been proximity to a cell tower. We had to know.

We were far from expert, but did know a few things about these fields that caused us concern. The electric service to and in our homes creates both magnetic fields from the flow of current and electrical fields as lines get energized by current. Utility lines and transformers, wiring faults, and any device powered by electricity will create magnetic fields of varying intensity. Electrical fields, which are more difficult to measure, are produced by the flow of current across lines, like those to lamps or appliances or through extension cords. Wi-Fi routers, smart meters, cell phones and cell phone transmitters are typical sources of radio frequencies and microwaves we encounter in our environment.

With each of these frequencies, the strength of the field typically diminishes quite quickly as you move away from the source. It is prolonged exposure to one or more of these frequencies at close range that research suggests — and this remains a highly contentious subject among the providers of services, the scientific community, and government regulators — may have harmful health impacts. Both electrical and magnetic fields can disrupt the deep sleep we need to repair and regenerate our bodies. Wi-Fi signals may have a similar effect. The two-way radio function of cell phones, based on microwaves, is not unlike a microwave oven — it heats up the brain when the phone is held to the ear. Research suggests that non-thermal radiation from pulsed signals found in appliances such as digital baby monitors, digital enhanced cordless communications (DECT) phones, and smart meters may also be disruptive at a cellular level.

Barbara had encountered patients at the Environmental Health Center who were so susceptible to electromagnetic frequencies (EMF) that they could only do testing and treatments in a room illuminated by daylight, with all electrical circuits turned off. One patient had to wear a tinfoil 'helmet' and gloves to protect herself from exposure to EMF. Another was so sensitive that the only place she could sleep was the back seat of her car. Barbara was certainly vulnerable to EMF, but not to this extent. For us, mitigation involved getting rid of the more obvious offenders in our life — the electric blanket, clock radio, and extension cords near the bed. Cell phone use was limited to headphone or hands-free functions, and we kept them out of the bedroom at night.

We found two reputable inspectors, who took about five hours to do their evaluation of our prospective purchase. The physical inspection confirmed what we sensed during our walk-throughs of the townhouse: it was a well-built home with a few easily corrected deficiencies. The other technician, who was measuring electromagnetic and radio fields, found a very different situation. While the house did not have higher-than-average levels of radio frequencies, there were major swings in the readings of EMF from room to room and along the hallways.

The strength of electromagnetic fields is measured in milliGauss (mG) by, ideally, a tri-axial Gaussmeter. (Quantifying electrical fields is more difficult and requires specialized equipment.) The World Health Organization recommends an average exposure to electromagnetic fields of no more than 3-4 mG for adults. The BioInitiative Report, a consortium of international experts on EMF and cell phone radiation, suggests a maximum prolonged exposure of about 1 mG. The German Institute for Baubiologie believes electromagnetic fields should be less than 0.2 mG for a healthy living environment.

Our consultant found spikes of between 20 mG and 40 mG in several places in the house. The master bedroom averaged about 4 mG, with the digital cordless phone in the dressing room recording a (literally) hair-raising 99 mG. The kitchen island, which was about five feet away from the refrigerator-freezer, measured about 5 mG when the compressors were running. It was becoming clear that this house, as it was, would not support Barbara's healing journey, which at the time was beginning to gather some positive momentum.

Still, we loved the house. We decided to see if the EMF issues could be "fixed." I contacted the local utility company, Oncor, thinking that the pole-mounted transformer might be emitting large amounts of radiation. They came out the next day and took measurements at the transformer and at various distances closer to the house. There was nothing out of the ordinary. In fact, a measurement taken 20 feet from the pole registered only 2.5 mG.

Undaunted, we hired an electrical contractor, Bob Owens, who had been recommended to us as experienced in helping homeowners mitigate issues with electromagnetic fields, an adjunct to his regular commercial and industrial work. During the inspection, he noted that the low-voltage, transformer-driven lighting in many of the rooms was raising the overall EMF, but he couldn't account for the spikes in his readings. He checked the wiring in the three- and four-way switches, appliances under load and the wiring in the main panel — nothing obviously out of spec. And with nothing capable of being isolated, there was really nothing to fix.

Perhaps a little embarrassed by his inability to find tangible answers, Bob proposed we turn off the main breaker to the house and re-measure. To everyone's bafflement, since there was no electrical current on in the house, the Gaussmeter continued to display readings above 5 mG. The only explanation we could come up with — and it was pure speculation — was that grounded electricity was possibly being attracted to underground watercourses and concentrating there. We really had no idea. But we were clear on one thing: we could not live in this house without potential danger to our health. We withdrew our offer and forfeited the $1,000.

(Following this experience, we bought a tri-axial Gaussmeter so we could do our own measurements before making an offer on a property. I found it on eBay, for about $230, offered by a seller who specialized in "ghost hunting" equipment. It has been a great investment, though it has yet to identify any ghosts. It did confirm the excellent EMF 'signature' of the house we eventually bought in Dallas, and we still carry it with us when we travel to find electromagnetic 'hot spots' in hotel rooms.)

Barbara's healing is not over, and perhaps never will be. We've offered this glimpse into her journey so far because knowing one's self, and acting consistently from that knowledge, was central to the success of the entire *+House* project. Barbara struggled for years to learn about and improve her health. We weren't about to squander all the work, time and money we had invested by leaving the decisions on building materials and processes entirely to those who had not shared our deep experience or necessary concern.

The truth is, once you've seen, you can't go back to blindness without a willful disregard for reality. We were not always clear about the detailed picture of our home's construction, but we knew that out-gassing chemicals in our environment, as well as the EMF profile of the house, had to be as close to zero as possible. Barbara's courage to question the status quo from the standpoint of what products and processes were best for her health — and the support we got in that exploration from the architects, contractor, and trades we worked with — was critically important to the outcome. As the following pages tell, our naïve questions led to some serendipitous and challenging evolution as the design took on form, yet always moved us closer to the healthy, sustainably built house we originally intended.

I want to emphasize, again, that our intention was uniquely ours. We informed it with the specifics of Barbara's various sensitivities, the opinions of others we respected, and most certainly a handful of personal beliefs. To us, it was ensuring that we created a living environment that supported our 'will to health' — to a life worth living.

Ours is not a journey that all individuals with health concerns will have the need, desire, or resources to follow. That's why the admonition to "know yourself" is essential to the overall success of whatever path you choose to follow. A new, healthier home may be exactly what you need. But it is equally likely that you may only need to create a healthier environment in the home you have. In either case, the lessons that follow will provide useful information for the intention you create.

Notes

1   Jenkins, McKay. *What's Gotten into Us: Staying Healthy in a Toxic World*. New York: Random House, 2011, p.13.

2   "The government isn't protecting you from dangerous chemicals. Congress must fix that." *The Washington Post*, May 24, 2016.

3   See also "The Hazards Lurking at Home: Top 10 Common Household Toxins" in *Time* magazine, April 1, 2010: **http://content.time.com/time/specials/packages/article/0,28804,1976909_1976895_1976914,00.html**

4   According to multiplechemicalsensitivity.org, an advocacy group, this health issue can be defined as follows: "Multiple Chemical Sensitivity; in broad terms it means an unusually severe sensitivity or allergy-like reaction to many different kinds of pollutants, including solvents, VOC's (Volatile Organic Compounds), perfumes, petrol, diesel, smoke, "chemicals" in general, and often encompasses problems with regard to pollen, house dust mites, and pet fur and dander... unlike true allergies—where the underlying mechanisms of the problem are relatively well understood and widely accepted, [MCS] is generally regarded as "idiopathic"— meaning that it has no known mechanism of causation and its processes are not fully understood."

5   Quoted in "Is It Safe to Play Yet," Michael Tortorello, *New York Times*, March 14, 2012.

6   From a lecture by Dr. Nagy to the University of Pennsylvania Medical School, February 6, 2012. Available at: **http://www.lisanagy.com**.

7   You can find the Exposure History Form at: **https://www.atsdr.cdc.gov/csem/exphistory/docs/CSEMExposHist-26-29.pdf**

Lesson 2:

Work with Accomplices You Trust

The downward health spiral that can result from chemical or electromagnetic exposures and the often lengthy, arduous climb back to health confounds most of us who have never been personally afflicted. How do we support those we care about without either personal experience or knowledge of the scientific evidence? Medical doctors without an understanding of environmental medicine usually focus on relieving the patient's symptoms. They typically remain uninformed of the underlying causes and their potential to result in chronic health issues. Patients themselves may be unaware of what affects their physical and mental well-being. Rather than being an understanding and accepting support system, some families can become passively hostile, particularly if the patient was formerly a high-functioning individual. Being confronted with the default reaction of "it's all in your head" is a common experience for many who struggle for answers.

If you're considering creating a healthy living environment out of necessity, you have likely encountered these attitudes in one form or another. We certainly have. It is why many environmentally sensitive individuals feel the need to be evangelical in communicating about their issues: it's an amalgam of wake-up call and basic self-protection. Too few people understand the dangers of exposure to toxic chemicals and electromagnetic radiation to themselves, let alone to those who, like Barbara, may have physical conditions that predispose them to be susceptible. Without at least some broad information about the problem, most people are unwilling to adjust their worldviews to accommodate the possibility that others may be affected by what they can't see, or which doesn't affect them in obvious ways.

This was an important realization for us at the beginning of the *+House* project. If we were going to be successful in creating a home that was also healthy, we understood that we bore a large part of the responsibility for educating the architects, contractor, trades, and even suppliers in our specific needs in that healthy environment. For their part, people working for us needed not only to be expert in their trades but also open to embracing our health issues — or at least their importance to us. As Barbara succinctly put it, "we need to find people who are open to the possibility that I experience life differently."

In the fall of 2009, we set to work assembling our team.

The Design Team

Compared to most people undertaking a custom building project, we began ours with a huge advantage. Our sister-in-law is Marianne McKenna, one of Canada's leading architects and a founding partner of Kuwabara Payne McKenna Blumberg Architects in Toronto. Marianne has designed and directed a wide range of acclaimed projects in the spheres of culture, business, and education. Given her workload, we were very grateful that she was willing to take on a key role in the design phase of our house. She wouldn't take charge of the design, but would ensure that the architects we hired were reputable, creative and, most importantly, willing to embrace Barbara's need for a clean living environment.

Marianne had in mind a small and highly regarded design studio in Toronto known as Superkül Architects to handle the design, materials and supervision for our project. Superkül was founded in 2002 by André D'Elia and Meg Graham, both former associates at Kuwabara Payne McKenna Blumberg and now partners in work and life. They had already garnered substantial praise for their work. While Superkül had a broad portfolio of project types, we were particularly impressed by their innovative urban and cottage residences, often built on challenging sites. One, an island retreat in Georgian Bay on eastern Lake Huron, blended the strong graphic lines of the house to the dramatic, wind-sculpted landscape of the Bay. It was a very creative marriage of form and context, just like our site would require.

Our initial meeting with André and Marianne took place at the property in late September 2009. Dressed in the architect's requisite black, with a shaved head and penetrating eyes, we found André immediately likeable. He had an easy-going manner that rode comfortably on what we perceived as a deep intensity of purpose to not only get the project right for us, but to make a statement about contemporary design outside the urban environment.

It didn't take all of us very long to arrive at a consensus on the existing house. While the property was exceptional — the former owners had transformed a forest of cedar and pine into a wonderland of manicured gardens and specimen trees — the house was beyond renovating. The footprint wouldn't allow for the scale of open spaces we envisioned overlooking a large pond, the property's central feature. The lower level was insufficiently damp-proofed to prevent continuing mold growth — a major health issue for anyone. And an indoor oil tank and furnace would slowly poison Barbara. We agreed that it was best to raze the structure, rip out the foundations and begin anew.

Then we laid out the real challenge: Design us a contemporary home on a demanding site and ensure that it will not make Barbara sick when we move in. And deal with multiple levels of government, including the notoriously difficult escarpment commission and water conservation authority, to get the required permits for siting, scope, and construction. There was a lengthy discussion of our health issues and of the books

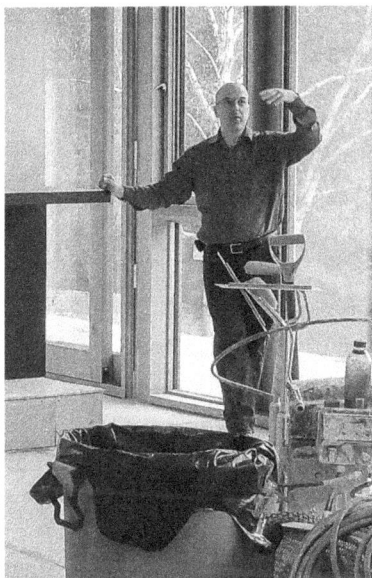

André D'Elia, the lead architect, explains a finishing detail later in the project.

that would be required reading, among them *Prescriptions for a Healthy House* and *Green Design: A Healthy Home Handbook*. We felt a genuine empathy in how André listened intently and asked thoughtful questions about our issues and objectives. He seemed enthusiastic about success and loved the location. And Superkül had Marianne's confidence. She knew their work ethic and design sensibility. We asked for a proposal, knowing without saying that we were unlikely to ask another architectural firm to bid.

Still, we had some apprehension. We wondered what André was really thinking about a project like ours. It would not be simple to execute properly more than an hour and a half from his office in the city. Barbara was concerned that he — or any architect, for that matter — wouldn't take her health issues fully to heart. Would he really seek out the best materials and advocate on our behalf with the contractor? Did he truly understand the seriousness of getting it right? Though we were fairly comfortable with André based on that first meeting, we were just as new to this from a building standpoint as he was. We would have to trust him.

When we later asked André about what he thought of the challenge of designing a contemporary home that is also healthy, he said, "I had an idea of what a healthy home was, but when I read the book [*Prescriptions for a Healthy House*] it changed a bit. I began to understand that there was a lot more information out there than I was aware of. I was really looking forward to the challenge because I knew it would be a huge learning experience.

"When we first started I talked to some colleagues about this project, about the challenges, one of them said, 'Don't you find that terrifying? What if it isn't healthy?' Because it is a prototype house. My comment was that it's kind of a numbers game. We're striving for 100 percent, but is that achievable? Probably not. We were going for the greatest percentage. That was the challenge, and I was excited by it. I was never in doubt or thought we couldn't do it. I always felt it would be successful."

In addition to the typical items like scope of work, phases of the project, estimated costs and fees, and a general schedule included in the proposal we received a week after our initial meeting, Superkül included a concise project description:

The project involves: the design of a new +/- 2,400 square-foot residence; landscape design immediately adjacent to the house, and renovation of the existing garage. The design of the house will incorporate green and passive strategies aimed at greater energy efficiency. The materials and products specified and the building construction techniques used will be chosen for their impact on the indoor air quality and on your environmental sensitivities.

It closely described our overall objective. Barbara and I signed the contract on October 2, 2009, and the design of +*House* finally began to move forward.

The Construction Team

In late January, 2010, we made the trip from Dallas to Toronto to begin the lengthy process of vetting materials and to interview potential builders. André had arranged for us to meet with the owners of two highly regarded construction firms, both of whom had built homes for Superkül clients. The contractors' websites were galleries of award-winning contemporary projects, all much grander and more costly than our own would be. We wanted to be assured that we would get the attention to detail and unrelenting oversight we knew would be essential for a small, prototype home like ours.

Both contractors expressed openness to the idea of building healthy, but seemed skeptical that our requirements could be met exactly. We gave each one *Prescriptions* and were adamant that, if selected, they would agree to follow the processes and materials it outlined to the letter. We spoke of Barbara's health issues and how even minor deviations or shortcuts could cause potentially serious problems for her. We talked about our commitment to using as many local trades, suppliers, and materials as possible. We knew we had to be evangelical about what we wanted, and perhaps annoyingly so.

That was a perception we could live with. Despite the stringent rules of engagement, both builders seemed interested in the challenge but were concerned about the potential cost of building a prototype home.

Ultimately, we chose Wilson Project Management. Their percentage fee on the total cost of the house construction and garage renovation was an attractive proposition we could get our minds around. While Wilson was based in Toronto, it had an office in Collingwood, Ontario, thirty minutes from our property. We were relieved to know that we would have a Collingwood-based site supervisor dedicated to our project — essential in our minds because we would be in Dallas during much of the building. And having built demanding contemporary houses around the province, Wilson had access to excellent trades and suppliers, both locally and in Toronto. Besides, Richard Wilson's wife had suffered from a mold-related illness, so we felt he would be sensitive to our issues. But, like our choice of architects, it took a lot of questioning, and eventually a leap of faith based on gut instinct.

We worked through the winter and spring with Superkül and Wilson's costing department to come up with a plan that would get us the quality of living environment we wanted at a price we could afford. Both teams fully embraced the ideas laid out in *Prescriptions for a Healthy House*, but we knew that good contemporary design, with its quality finishes and custom installations, would not be inexpensive. While the additional costs of healthy construction were simply an unknown to us as clients, we expected a final tally a little under $1 million.

At more than double what we had in mind, the first budget for the concept we provisionally approved took our breath away. Surely there were some crazy assumptions or input errors on the spreadsheet. It reminded us of the quip we often heard from friends who knew we were building: "How much will it cost to build a new house? Get three estimates and add them together." During the subsequent rounds of 'value engineering' the design program changed significantly — smaller footprint, single story, fewer retaining walls — but still kept the essential character and healthy materials we wanted. We resigned ourselves to a more modest house, a decision we regretted throughout the construction but came to appreciate when we finally moved in (and finished paying the bills).

Behind the scenes at Wilson, budgeting for a healthy project, we later learned, was anything but straightforward. Dyson Simpson, who had the responsibility of pricing our job, felt that the overriding difference between conventional construction and the healthy mandate was never being able to make airtight assumptions about what would work.

"I do budgets all the time," he said, "and I make assumptions everywhere, but they turn out to be pretty accurate because I know from other projects how much things are going to cost. But when you deal with a healthy house, you start from scratch. It's the same process, but you go about doing things differently. You spend less time doing square footages and plugging in numbers that we have from past experience. You're more cautious about numbers, and you rely more on quotes and actual figures from experts in the field.

"Another dynamic of the project was that you were more hands-on in the budget phase, because a lot of decisions that would typically come into play later on in the project were made at the budget phase. We had to decide which road to go down with certain kinds of products. The question was always, how far were we willing to go and at what cost? That all had to be established at the budget stage, which was a real challenge, mostly for you."

Why for us? Because we were the final arbiters of the delicate balance between healthy and practical, and between nice-to-have and must-have. It's a balance founded on knowing yourself — on an honest assessment of your needs and your resources. If there are trade-offs to be made, keep focused on your intention to health.

Richard Wilson assigned Jeff Pepper to the job of site supervisor and gave him full responsibility for every aspect of the construction: hiring trades, ordering materials, managing the site, and staying within budget. In keeping with the learning curve that everyone on the project was experiencing, it was Jeff's introduction to healthy building. With twenty-five years of building and carpentry experience, he was hardly a neophyte. Jeff operates with a casual, friendly manner that complements his quick mind and deep well of real-world construction knowledge. And at six-foot-four and about two hundred and twenty pounds, he's also an imposing presence. It seemed a perfect combination in someone charged not just with laying down the health laws on our site, but keeping the whole enterprise on time and to a tight budget.

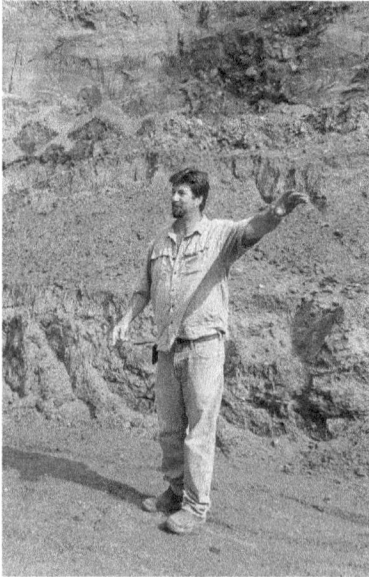

Jeff Pepper, our construction supervisor, directing the excavation of the site.

Even with all his experience, the project was unnerving for Jeff. He told us, "I remember the day I was onsite and Barbara handed me "The Book." I started reading and thought, oh my god, concrete: what's fly ash? And that's just one product. I didn't know the extent of the challenges in the house initially. Then every single day it was the same question: where's the potential problem for Barbara?

"I think the pretty much full-time site management on the project was the biggest difference between it and conventional construction. With some projects, we budget part-time supervision on processes like drywall. But on your home, there were such strict guidelines on materials and cleanup that we had to ensure any issues would get dealt with quickly."

Jeff and the rest of the team took on each challenge with what seemed to us as equanimity and interest. Because they had our trust — much of our communication took place by email and photos — we left them to make most of the daily decisions as they saw fit. They knew our budget. We expected them to help us stay within it unless we made a deliberate decision to add cost in return for a real benefit, which we did on several occasions. What bound us, beyond the client-supplier relationship, was the common intention to create something great and healthy. We were confident that both Wilson and Superkül would fight the inertia of the status quo to protect Barbara's health, and our confidence was rewarded time and again. They displayed a willingness to trust in the process of finding the right answers when nothing seemed to be right. It felt like a great collaboration, even from afar.

There Will Be Resistance

Common intention or not, the building of *+House* was not all 'light and love' for Jeff Pepper and Wilson. While all the trades and suppliers selected by Wilson were exceptionally competent, their very success occasionally presented an initial stumbling block for a demanding construction process like ours. After all, they built their reputations using certain products and ways of doing things. It was difficult for some to question the status quo, especially for health issues that they may not have fully understood and never encountered in a client before.

We had lived through the trouble that can come from not being very clear and very direct with trades about our health concerns. In 2008, we intended to re-carpet the master bedroom in our Dallas condo. With Barbara going through the worst of her testing protocol at the Environmental Health Center, we were very careful to find and order an organic wool carpet manufactured with neutral backing and formaldehyde-free glue. The extra expense of the carpet and shipping from a supplier in California would be worth the cost.

Because I would be out of town visiting a client and Barbara was undergoing testing that day, we arranged with a young designer who had helped us furnish the apartment to oversee the carpet installation. Absolutely no glues, we said. Only tackless carpet strips around the perimeter of the room.

Barbara awoke in the middle of the night with a nauseous headache and the smell of toxic glue permeating the room. The installers evidently defaulted to their preferred method or had perhaps run into a problem they were not creative enough to solve in a healthier way. Maybe it was passive resistance to us telling them how to install carpet. In any case, Barbara moved to the living room and got what sleep she could. In the morning, in a call I'm sure the designer will not forget, she demanded that the carpet be removed that day and all the glue be scraped from the floor.

Barbara headed back to the Health Center for another difficult day of testing. She met with Carolyn Gorman, a consultant at the Center and author of the book *Less-Toxic Alternatives*. In her view, if the glue couldn't be completely removed, which appeared to be the case, the best solution was to cover the entire floor in heavy-duty tinfoil, like might be used to line the bottom of an oven. Then the seams would have to be sealed with aluminum tape, effectively containing the off-gassing glue. For someone like Barbara, already feeling horribly sick from the combination of testing and chemicals, it was a tedious and miserable job and she let me know it. But it worked reasonably well until we eventually covered the floor, tinfoil and all, with inert cork.

Experiences like this made us determined to be very clear about our needs in the building of +*House*. We presented it as a challenge to both Superkül and Wilson. Could they keep themselves, and everyone they worked with on the project, deeply and professionally committed to getting as healthy an outcome as possible?

André's view of the healthy building process was, "Basically, you need to be open-minded. People are used to doing things in a certain way, and it's difficult to get them to change that. You can still maintain the same process, but you need to be aware of materials. You tend to fall back on materials you've had success with, and when you don't know them [healthy building options] it involves more research and more time. You have to see it as a challenge, as a great opportunity. You have to be enthusiastic."

Jeff explained the challenge of building a prototype house as it related to the window supplier. Windows were a major component of the design and construction of +*House*, spanning nearly ninety feet across the south side of the house to a height of fourteen feet. "Look at it from the supplier's perspective," he said. "He's already offering a high-quality product. He's thrilled with his epoxy finish, with all the chemicals in it, because it's worked for twenty years. So he'll give a warranty on that. Then we come along, really good clients of his, and say he has to use this Safecoat product he's never heard of. He wasn't thrilled with it, and it was a challenge to use in his spraying equipment, but he still did a great job."

Our requirements for the electrical system were another issue for the trades. Because of our sensitivities to electromagnetic fields, we required the finished house to have an average reading of .75 milliGauss or less. (Recall that "MilliGauss" is a measure of electromagnetic field, or EMF, strength.) One candidate for the job said, "No way, a hairdryer will blow that out." When they learned that their work would be subject to very strict specifications and measurement — the test at the end of the course — several others refused to even quote.

The electricians did succeed in delivering a house with an average EMF reading even lower than we specified, but not without some unnerving moments before the final connections were made and power turned on. As Jeff recalled, "You gave me the Gauss meter, but without electricity hooked up, we didn't know. But it's still my responsibility. We did everything in shielded cable that we thought was going to be close to the living areas, but was it going to make a difference? I didn't know. I walked around the site office with the meter. I took it home. The electrician took it home to measure his own house and said, '.75 milliGauss or better? Are you kidding?'"

The concrete mix and concrete troweling for the heated slab were also a source of much resistance. We will deal with issue of the concrete mix and its finishing in Lesson 4, but the push-back we received on the troweling technique was directly related to the healthy building mandate. Since the concrete pour was taking place in January, the building envelope had to be sealed for the electric heaters to maintain the temperature required to cure the concrete. All the bids specified gas-powered trowelers for the pour. We wouldn't take the health risk of having residue from gas exhaust trapped inside the house, and we insisted on the use of an electric model. But the supplier being considered by Wilson had built his reputation on using a gas-powered trowel. As he said to Jeff in an email, "I just talked to a finisher friend of mine. He has used electric trowels before but says they don't work that well. Would not recommend it for this application at all. It will have to be gas-powered trowels."

Rather than lose the job, the supplier relented and eventually delivered an excellent product without compromising the healthy mandate. But we had to insist on what we needed, and he had to be willing to step out of his comfort zone. There was learning on both sides.

THIS IS A HEALTHY HOUSE ONLY SPECIFIED PRODUCTS & PROCEDURES ALLOWED.

TOXIC SUBSTANCES INCLUDING PESTICIDES, FUNGICIDES, NOXIOUS CLEANING PRODUCTS ARE PROHIBITED. GASOLINE-GENERATED MACHINES OR OPEN COMBUSTION HEATERS SHALL NOT BE USED INSIDE THE HOUSE.

SMOKING AT CONSTRUCTION SITE PROHIBITED.

SPILLS OF FUELS, SOLVENTS OR CHEMICALS MUST BE AVOIDED. ALTERNATIVES TO SPECIFIED MATERIALS MUST BE APPROVED IN WRITING PRIOR TO USE BY OWNER AND/OR ARCHITECT.

The use of substances listed below is prohibited:

1. *Herbicides, fungicides, insecticides and other pesticides, except as specified*

2. *Composite wood products containing urea formaldehyde binders*

3. *Asphalt or products containing asphalt or bitumen*

4. *Commercial cleaning products other than those specified*

5. *Adhesives, paints, sealers, stains and other finishes except as specified*

6. *Any building materials contaminated by mold or mildew*

7. *Any building materials or components that have been contaminated while in storage or during shipment*

As clients, we had become aware of our own resistance to change. When Barbara began working with Dr. Rea at the Environmental Health Center in Dallas, he asked if she liked to cook. "Sure," she said, "we cook most nights." "Bet you have a gas range," he replied. "You need to get rid of it." We loved that gas range and its ease of use; we literally couldn't imagine how we'd go back to electric. It was another year before Barbara realized how ill the products of combustion from the gas made her feel. Despite having just completed an extensive renovation of the kitchen, we reluctantly installed a flat-top electric range that turned out to be more than acceptable for our level of skill.

That's the lesson in resistance: if you're open to honest examination of where you're digging in your heels, it gives you an opportunity to re-imagine what's possible. A willingness to be flexible is a useful character trait.

Clear Responsibilities

Aside from paying the bills, our primary responsibility as owners throughout the design and construction of *+House* was to make the communication of our health issues, design preferences, and choice of materials as clear as possible. Barbara and I wanted to be heard; in fact, we *had* to be heard. We used books such as *Prescriptions for a Healthy House*, *Green Design: A Healthy Home Handbook* and *Homes That Heal* to convey the general principles of healthy building and provide guidance on materials. We were actively involved with the architects on their specification of materials. Barbara 'sniff-tested' almost every material that went into the house to gauge her reaction. We questioned choices of products and processes. We researched material safety data sheets whenever there was concern about potential toxicity.

There was more to this than getting the healthiest materials possible. It also entailed fairness to the trades bidding to work on the project and the impact of our choices on the budget. As Jeff Pepper put it when asked about push-back from trades on using the materials we needed: "We'd have to specify a material, do the contract, then 'phone our trade' because a lot of them signed up with the original set of blueprints. We didn't know whether some materials would work. Then, when we finally knew the specifics, we redid the contracts and tried to keep it within the budget or let you know that it was going to be a little more money. So the trades were well aware of what was coming, and you had the chance to make those decisions."

It says a great deal about the quality of the tradespeople selected by Wilson that, despite some uncertainty around materials or processes, no one ever walked off the job because they were unable to make the transition to new ways of building. Everyone seemed to appreciate the opportunity to work on a prototype house, learn new perspectives on building, and make a little money along the way. Nor did they want to alienate an important contractor like Wilson.

In other words, the trades were professional. Indeed, that was *their* responsibility: to be expert craftspeople disciplined in delivering their product according to the needs or demands of the client. In our case, part of Wilson's mandate, in collaboration with the architect, entailed vetting the trades for us. Not just for suitability, but for attitude toward the idea of creating a healthy house. Superkül established the ground rules early in the process with a statement[1] that appeared on each page of the working drawings (see box).

Speaking of resistance, a note on cigarettes. Smoking is a habit of choice for some people, but it is not our choice and it is not a healthy choice. We insisted that there be no smoking on site at any time or during any phase of the construction, from excavation to finish carpentry. If they needed a smoke break, everyone walked 180 feet to the road, sometimes grudgingly. Especially the roof and deck framers, who often worked in the rain and didn't understand why they couldn't smoke in open air. We understood their reluctance, but saying yes to smoking would have compromised the integrity of the healthy house idea, and possibly led to more serious compromises. The trades had to know they were part of the total healthy building solution. Clear guidelines were essential, along with the credibility that came from consistent enforcement on the site.

Other Accomplices

While the architects, contractor and trades had the most prominent roles in the success of +*House*, many other professionals played parts integral to the outcome. Some were obvious choices from the beginning, but others had more to do with what seemed to be chance than careful planning. That was another important lesson for us. Questioning the status quo and staying open to new ideas from unexpected sources not only resulted in a much healthier house, it also saved money and reduced our impact on the environment.

These accomplices fell into three broad categories: the necessary, the serendipitous, and the unwitting.

The necessary accomplices were much as we expected. The soil engineers who tested the quality of the local soil, its ability to bear the footings for the foundation, and the requirements for retaining the hill behind the house. The structural engineers, who on several occasions had to rework their calculations to deal with new and unusual building materials. The electrical engineers, who ensured that the lighting and wiring runs were not just efficient but reduced electromagnetic radiation to as low a level as possible. And there was the millwork team led by Andy Johnston, who worked almost as long at his computer trying to find the right combination of products and sealants as he did actually making and installing the cabinetry.

We will have much more to say about the serendipitous accomplices we encountered in Lesson 3 and Lesson 4, but they brought tremendous value to the entire project. In mid-2010, for example, Barbara and I visited EcoInhabit (ecoinhabit.com), a store in Meaford, Ontario that offers green building products, eco books, and construction services. Our mission was simply to see the store and find out if Wilson could order Safecoat products through them. During our visit, one of the staff introduced us to a product called American Clay as an alternative to paint, and we were greatly impressed with its texture, colors and potential health benefits. During the conversation, staff also highly recommended two men to us as consultants. The first, Robert Stellar, was a local healthy building expert — we had no idea there was such a profession — who a few weeks later would become a major influence on the construction materials we used. The second was Tim Singbeil, the owner of EcoInhabit, who ultimately erected the foundation and walls of +*House*.

As the dimensions and siting of the house began to take shape, we brought in a local landscape architect to develop a preliminary landscape plan required by the Niagara Escarpment Commission and the local conservation authority, which oversees watercourses and wetlands. Given the issues of slope and drainage, we thought the money spent for drawings from a licensed professional was worthwhile. We made it very clear that budget was an issue — a perception reinforced by Wilson and Superkül — and that we wanted a natural approach to the landscape rather than the formal gardens that surrounded the former house.

Months passed. When the plan finally arrived, it included a massive stone and wire mesh 'gabion' wall across the back hill, well over one hundred feet of reinforced concrete wall spanning the front of the house, extensive plantings and a budget more than twice what we had expected. The designer would not substantially alter his plan, so we paid the invoice and looked for alternatives. As Lesson 8 discusses, they came in the form environmentally friendly retaining 'bags' at the base of the back hill, organic compost on the front hill and the decision to remove all the hardscape from the driveway. Our former landscape architect, who claimed to prefer natural landscapes, actually became an unwitting accomplice in the creation of a sustainable landscape design that added a handful of LEED points to the overall total.

Notes

1   Adapted from *Prescriptions for a Healthy House*, 3rd Edition.

Lesson 3:

Good Design Can Be Healthy Design

I am always amazed at my own willful disregard of evident facts in the face of my own desire to do, or have, something. I can think of all manner of ill-premised decisions that came back to vex me, from cars to relationships.

Convincing ourselves that we could live in the country house we had just purchased in Mulmur, even for one summer, was one of those decisions.

When I first inspected the house the previous November, there was an obvious musty smell in the bedroom of the walkout basement — typically, a sure sign of mold growth. When we returned late the following January for our pre-closing inspection, the odor remained, even after months of winter heating. Still, we went ahead with the closing, knowingly overlooking the mold issue. The house would be coming down, after all. Surely we could get the mold remediated before we moved in for the summer. We should have known much better. We had already had an experience that would be a major influence on the design of the healthy house we intended to build.

One day in 2007, I opened the master bedroom linen closet of our home in Carmel to find a distinct musty smell. I had spent enough time in damp Ontario basements growing up to know there was mold growing somewhere. There it was on the ceiling, a telltale gray etching on the drywall, the result, we discovered, of a small leak around a vent stack protruding through the roof. It was a very upsetting discovery for Barbara. She had learned just weeks before that she had already been exposed to a mold toxic to her kidneys. Now her sanctuary had been invaded.

We moved out to the guest room and in moved the environmental consultants to capture interior and exterior air samples, do moisture mapping and take swabs to determine mold spore concentrations. The dismaying verdict concluded that we had an "indoor fungal reservoir." Worse, the testing revealed the primary mold was *Stachybotrys*, often described as the highly toxic "black mold." The basement in Mulmur smelled just like it.

Commons molds like *Stachybotrys atra* and *Aspergillis fumigatus*, left unchecked, can lead to many kinds of health issues. According to both the Centers for Disease Control and Prevention and the Environmental Protection Agency in the United States, molds — whether the spores are living or dead — can produce a wide variety of allergic reactions such as skin rashes, runny noses, wheezing, and even asthma. For people with compromised or suppressed immune systems, like Barbara, the effects of inhaling mycotoxins produced by molds can be extremely serious. Prolonged exposures can lead to acute or chronic liver damage or chronic central nervous system damage — even cancer.[1]

It was no surprise then that the remediation professionals in California had a lot of respect for the *Stachybotrys* they encountered in our closet. Dressed head to toe in white hazmat suits and wearing half-mask respirators, they sealed off the master bedroom, covered and taped the furniture and created negative air pressure to siphon air (and spores) from the room to the outside. All materials they removed were sealed in special hazardous material bags, lowered to the ground and taken away for incineration. Industrial HEPA air filters ran for weeks. A second air quality test indicated normal spore counts — counts at about the same concentration as the outside air — but a visual inspection revealed mold stains on the rafters. We consulted with Carolyn Gorman at the Environmental Health Center in Dallas. She was adamant that all traces of mold had to be removed lest it revitalize, and so we repeated the entire process. By the time our tiny closet ceiling was rid of the mold and repaired, three months — and thousands of dollars — had passed through our hands.

Unlike that closet ceiling, there was no visible mold growth on the walls in the dank, low-ceilinged basement of the Mulmur house. We knew whatever lurked down there must be dealt with professionally so we could get through the summer. We hired a well-regarded "disaster cleanup" company to seal off the lower level from the rest of the house, remove the carpet, sand off the carpet glue and swab the concrete floor, plasterboard walls and wood stairs. Their preferred chemical cleaner was chlorine-based. That would not work for Barbara. Besides, our research suggested that chlorine was an ineffective weapon against mold on all but hard, non-porous surfaces. It wouldn't work on the mycelia, or roots, that might have burrowed into the drywall or stairs. The remediation company found an alternative cleaner, but wouldn't guarantee their work. And we were packing the house in Carmel and getting ready to drive to Dallas. In other words, hardly in a position to monitor their efforts.

When we arrived to move in a few weeks later, the basement was more disaster than disaster cleaned up. The carpet and underpad had been glued to the concrete floor, and its removal had left behind tufts of foam padding that scraping and sanding had not removed. The wooden stairs were bare and stained. Worse, despite the remediation and cleanup, the musty smell was still obvious, but now redolent with an ugly chemical overtone.

Barbara couldn't go downstairs for more than a few minutes without the feeling of her chest tightening — a sure reaction to the mold in her case — and we did our best to try to keep the lower level sealed off with plastic sheeting. We brought back the mold specialists for another round of testing and air samples. Tests showed that the *Aspergillus* spores were elevated but not seriously so. The next step in remediation would require removing all the drywall to find out what, if anything, might be growing back there. That seemed an expensive strategy for a house we were intending to pull down. We borrowed a dehumidifier to dry out the area and when that proved insufficient, bought another fifty-liter unit. It was an almost impossible task to keep the basement dry. On particularly warm, humid days, we would have to empty both units every twenty-four hours.

We discovered that moisture, heat and mold go hand in hand if there is a growth medium — think of the scenes of mold growth in the flooded homes of New Orleans after Hurricane Katrina. Our mold issue appeared to come from a combination of the site and the construction of the house. Where the house was sited, the property rises more than fifty feet from the pond to the top of the hill and then continues upwards on a gentler grade to the back of the property. Building a tall, narrow house in this spot necessitated a massive reinforced concrete retaining wall as much as fifteen feet in height that partially wrapped around the east and west sides of the house. On much of the lower level, the concrete wall was exposed—it had never been properly finished. And while we could see that there was no evidence of water penetration, it took us some time to realize that the real culprit was condensation. When the humid summer air met the cold unfinished walls, the water vapor precipitated out of the air and gave the mold a perfect Petri dish in which to grow. That would be the major factor in our decision not to include a habitable lower level in whatever design we eventually chose to build.

"Have you ever been in a basement that didn't have some sort of problem with dampness?" asked Marianne McKenna, our consulting architect. We were discussing the overall design program for the house. "If you think about what a basement ends up being used for, it's against everything we're moving towards, which is to stop accumulating things we're not using. Unless you're trying to put people down there, which isn't a good idea in most cases."

She explained that in the 'old days' of house design a basement had to accommodate a furnace, oil tank and water heater. It provided thermal insulation and a frost barrier in cold climates. Now mechanical rooms are becoming smaller as technology drives innovation in furnaces and on-demand water heaters, and new materials provide better insulation against cold and water penetration. To build a full or partial basement, if not absolutely necessary, doesn't make much sense anymore. Worse, it invites the same mold issues with which we had been dealing.

Conceptually, we were fine without a basement, but we found it difficult to imagine what the overall design might look like. The site imposed some significant constraints. Building at the top of the hill to avoid moisture would have destroyed the relationship of the house to the pond and turned every trip from the garage uphill to the house into an athletic event. The obvious location, centered on the site of the existing house and retaining wall, had its own challenges. The available building area was just eighty feet deep, with the pond across its entire southern perimeter and a sharply rising hill to the north that shed large amounts of water during rains and the spring snow melt.

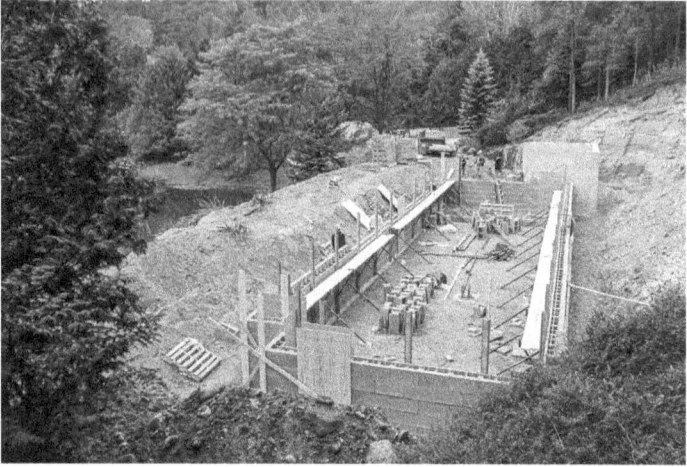

An extremely tight site on all four sides, with a narrow entrance from the road.

Additionally, mature specimen trees guarded access to this long, narrow strip of land, including five twenty-foot weeping Nootka cypress trees that would have to be relocated before construction began. The escarpment commission insisted on a ninety-foot setback from the pond in order to gain its approval — a virtually impossible demand to meet given the steep slope of the hill — but later relented due to the location of the existing house. For its part, the conservation authority wanted to ensure we would be above the flood plain of the pond, which had been the case for decades.

Ultimately, these physical challenges dictated the form of the house.

From Superkül's perspective, the healthy home mandate influenced construction but not necessarily the design. As project architect Geoff Moote put it, "We knew how the building should be sited, we knew how we wanted it to perform passively, in terms of cooling and how the light would enter the space. I don't think a healthy home can dictate form. It's really the building process and the research behind it that has the greatest influence.

"The biggest challenge of design was how that grade married with the house. Getting the floor slab at the right height. We looked at it extensively on the computer, then went to the site and looked some more. We couldn't really move the house back further into the hill and we didn't want it to be too low. It was quite a balancing act to get it right."

Initially, we weren't so sure they had got it right. As excavation proceeded, all our untrained eyes saw was a deep rectangular hole and a formerly pristine hillside that had been clawed away for safety during construction. A twelve-foot-high extension to the existing exterior retaining wall made sense to us; there was a lot of hill to hold back. But when the foundation walls went up nearly seven feet and then the entire structure was filled with earth for the concrete slab, we began to understand the space sacrifice and added cost that designing a healthier, mold-free house could entail. We had to trust that this was all in our best interests.

As part of our briefing to Superkül, we had written a few paragraphs about what we intended our new home to be. We told them, "The design will be modern as well as appropriate to the environment. The interior space should be open and flowing, with the master suite offering a place to 'get away,' if necessary. We want the home to be as energy-efficient as possible, within the bounds of budget and common sense. In the choice of materials, construction, finishes and furnishings, Barbara's sensitivity to chemicals must override budget as the primary concern."

There was one other thing: we wanted to bring the feeling of the outdoors — the beautiful pond and its surrounding gardens — into the house as a visual element in the overall design.

The first presentation of the schematic design concepts took place online between Toronto and Dallas in December 2009. The proposed house had everything we wanted. In fact, it had a lot more than we expected for the money we expected to spend. That disconnect later prompted us to consider making a recommendation to residential architects everywhere: consider running some preliminary budgets before presenting great plans to novice clients. It will save everyone the time and fees and heartache involved in the inescapable reengineering that reality usually imposes.

Still, the essential elements of the design were what we had in mind. Marianne's initial design concept positioned the house on the site, perpendicular to the road. It was her view that the house should have a feeling of "long and low" in its proportions, with a sequence of enfilade, or aligned, rooms that progressed from entry to guest room, to living space, and finally to the master bedroom suite. She envisaged a low-pitched roof to make the structure simple, as well as framing that would be repeatable across the 90-foot-south-facing façade. This front window wall, looking south over the pond, rose 14 feet in Superkül's design — ten-foot lift and slide glass doors with a three-foot clerestory above — would create our own wide-screen theatre of the outdoors. A generous deck would span the entire front of the house and wrap around the west side of the house, integrating the living space with the outdoors. The exterior structure would have to be reinforced concrete, clad in cedar. With the house embedded in the slope, Geoff explained, sustainable alternatives such as straw bale or rammed earth construction could not meet the tests of moisture protection or dimensional stability.

The plans proposed that a flat roof would drop gently from its high point on the south side to the lower north side of the house, a slope of about three feet. André and Geoff showed us computer studies detailing the effect of the roof overhang on the sun's penetration into the house at various times of the year — most in winter, least in summer. The design would allow us to take full advantage of natural light throughout the year while minimizing solar heat gain. Another element of the bioclimatic design was the use of cross-ventilation. The massive screened doors and smaller operating windows across the front of the house would open the house to breezes from the pond. Screened clerestory windows along the top of the north wall, three operating skylights and ceiling fans would encourage the flow of air through the house, keeping it comfortable on all but the hottest and most humid days. And that would help ensure the house was less likely to be subject to dust and mold.

We were delighted. Nature definitely had been given an open invitation to be part of our living environment.

Superkül proposed that the primary source of heating for the house be through a hydronic radiant heat system in the concrete slab. In hydronic systems, water circulates through linked polyethylene tubing set in the floor, and heat radiates upwards through convection. They're clean and, apart from the mechanical pumps required to move the water in the tubes, silent. The more typical forced-air system of heating, André believed, with its major ductwork and blowing air, was unacceptable for a healthy house design — too much potential for dust and discomfort. We liked the simplicity of a heated concrete floor and its health advantages, though we were skeptical about how comfortable it would be underfoot. We would probably need supplemental heat in winter but we could augment the floor by using the ventilation system to distribute heat from the electric furnace. A great idea in principle.

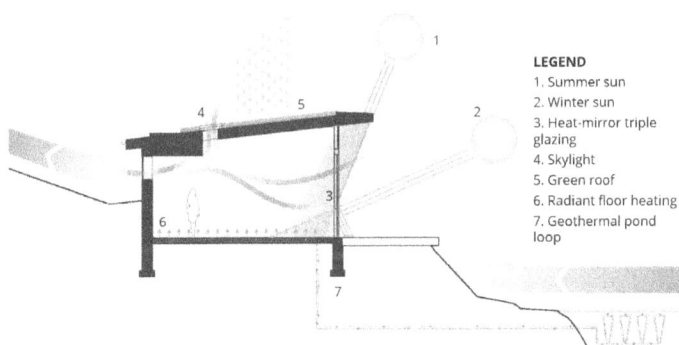

LEGEND
1. Summer sun
2. Winter sun
3. Heat-mirror triple glazing
4. Skylight
5. Green roof
6. Radiant floor heating
7. Geothermal pond loop

As André and Geoff explained it, the primary job of the ventilation system would be cooling. The ducts would be placed high on the walls to get an even distribution of falling cool air. In winter, supplemental heat from these ducts and rising heat from the slab could be mixed and circulated by the ceiling fans. A high volume of fresh air would be an important component of the health of the house, and not just from open windows and screened doors. A heat recovery ventilator (HRV) would run continually, taking in a large volume of outside air, conditioning it slightly, filtering out particulates and then pumping it through the distribution system. The exhaust would run constantly as well. Filtration would be handled by the hospital-grade Lifebreath whole house air cleaner, which would remove nearly one hundred percent of all allergens and pollutants through its combination of "turbulent flow precipitation" and a "high energy particulate air" (HEPA) filter.

All of this seemed like smart healthy house protocol to us. We knew that indoor air quality was a critical component of a healthy living environment; many homes have far higher concentrations of pollutants like dust, fibers, molds, and off-gasses than the outside air. Barbara and I needed as close to zero as possible.

Not content to let mechanical equipment take care of pollutants, Superkül envisioned the millwork — not designed at this point in the process — as contributing to the overall cleanliness of the house. The extensive millwork would be closed wherever possible. Open shelving would be kept to a minimum. The tops of closets and cupboards would be integrated into the walls, eliminating out-of-reach areas for dust to collect. The sealed concrete floor would be easy to vacuum or damp-mop.

What's more, the entire home would have a light, natural palette of materials. "We want the house to be comfortable," explained André. "We want it to be a home where you'll feel at ease, not on edge. Some of the problem with houses that are too modern is that you feel you can never really relax in them."

We were hooked. We gave Superkül the green light to develop the plans further. They would contact Wilson to begin a preliminary budget. It was tremendously exciting to see our ideas gain the momentum of manifestation. But as I would learn once again, you must take responsibility for what you bring into being.

The truth is that, throughout the planning process, we didn't have much in mind other than the 'nice-to-haves' of a house design. Being naturally client-centered, Superkül looked into our souls and crafted our wish list into what Meg Graham would later call "… a synthesis of healthy design, sustainability, and what is classically considered 'high design.'"

The initial plan was breathtaking to us. Twenty-seven hundred square feet of mostly open, soaring spaces. Superkül incorporated a narrow second story, cantilevered backwards, that seemed to rest barely supported on the hill behind. A dedicated yoga space for Barbara adjoined the generous master bedroom. A screened porch anchored the west end of the house and could be easily turned into another bedroom if required. An outdoor shower brought an exotic element to the forests of Mulmur. A second fireplace on one corner of the deck evoked long evenings of great conversation with friends around the fire. We created a space in our minds for our dream house and moved in.

Reality shattered our grand delusion in the form of the preliminary budget. It was more than twice what we had intended to spend, requiring us to become familiar with the term "value engineering." Over the next four or five revisions, the second story disappeared, the zinc roof became steel, the north wall of the house evolved into a retaining wall, the screened porch became a second bedroom and the footprint of the house shrunk to a little over twenty-one hundred square feet. Barb would have to do with a smaller yoga 'area.' And there would be no forest-view shower. Yet there was never a question about making the house as healthy as possible on the budget we had.

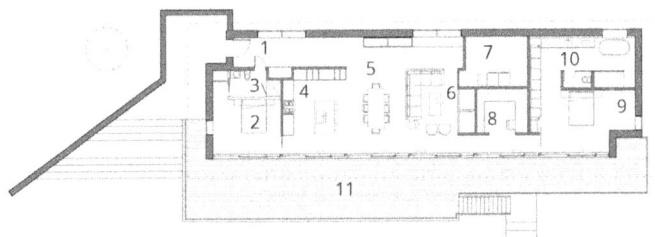

GROUND LEVEL PLAN

1. Entrance
2. Bedroom
3. Washoom
4. Kitchen
5. Dining area
6. Living room
7. Laundry
8. Study
9. Master bedroom
10. Master washroom
11. Outdoor terrace

N
0 5 10   20M

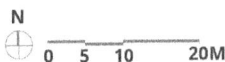

Superkül's final, as-built floor plan.

By the middle of May 2010, after many devoted hours of work by André and his team, we settled on a compromise design and a reasonable price. Superkül proceeded on the working drawings while Wilson negotiated with trades and suppliers to fine-tune the pricing. The weeping cypress trees were relocated and other species removed and sent to a nursery for storage. Habitat for Humanity picked the old house clean of its useful parts. Demolition was set to begin.

Just days before Superkül was to go to the county building department for the construction permits, we asked a simple question about reinforced concrete that brought everything to a complete halt and dramatically changed the primary materials to be used in the house. As we discovered to everyone's surprise, some aspects of the design and engineering were not as healthy as they could be. New plans would have to be drawn and new engineering opinions obtained before construction could proceed.

Notes

1   U.S. Environmental Protection Agency, "Mold Remediation in Schools and Commercial Buildings," Appendix B, 9/30/2010 Update.

Lesson 4:

Ask Questions Constantly

I assume you have read this far because you suspect that your home can make you sick — or worse, has already done so. Once you have arrived at that place in understanding, it's your responsibility to begin to question everything that goes into building, furnishing, and maintaining your home. That's as true of a renovation as it is of a new home.

That's why this chapter is titled "Ask Questions Constantly."

Given Barbara's sensitivity to environmental chemicals and her impaired ability to detoxify her body when she came in contact with them, we began by questioning most everything about the processes and materials that would be used in *+House*. We found many answers and valuable advice in *Prescriptions for a Healthy House*. But as thorough as it is, *Prescriptions* doesn't have every answer or the most current information on materials. And as skilled as our team was in their combined knowledge of materials and construction, answers to important questions eluded them from time to time. It was emphatically *not* because they did not care to know. Sometimes even experts don't know what questions to ask, a situation that can be exacerbated by a lack of understanding or information about a client's specific health issues.

That's why we had to advocate for ourselves throughout the process, despite the care and concern that was evident from everyone on the team. We became our own 'Environmental Protection Agency' because only we knew the personal health consequences of not doing so. Our questions must have sounded completely naïve on many occasions, and they probably were. But it was the willingness to question others' expertise and what they take for granted, as well as the courage not to compromise in the face of difficult and often technical decisions, that made a substantial difference in the success of the outcome. As this lesson shows, without constant questions our project might not have been as healthy as it could have been, despite hard work and good intentions on everyone's part.

Anyone going down a similar path will not have all the answers either, even with resources like this book and others in the bibliography. That's a good place to be. Our experience showed us that when we were in a state of *not* knowing — and living with the uncertainty until we found the answers we needed — everyone's learning accelerated.

By mid-June 2010, we had a design that met our goals for a healthy house at a price we could afford. With the major changes complete, everyone shifted into high gear to finalize the plans for presentation to the township and county building departments. By now we were at least a month behind schedule, and we wanted to get the construction back on track. Closing in the structure so that interior work could continue through the winter was an important milestone, at least in our minds.

It was about this time that the forces of serendipity intervened and set in motion a series of explorations that led to a substantial improvement in the healthy profile of the house. And to be fair to the many sensible decisions that had already been made, it also added unanticipated time, anxiety, and expense for everyone involved.

The evolution began with a simple question about a seemingly innocuous aspect of the construction process. I am reproducing much of the actual email thread here because it not only brings home the necessity of questioning the most basic procedures in building a healthy home, it also shows the limits of experience and expertise — and even the very best intentions — in building a prototype house.

On June 17th, Jeff Pepper, Wilson's site supervisor, wrote to Geoff Moote, the project architect, copying us:

> I am just putting in a little overtime trying to keep ahead of the project and I have been studying release agents from the *Healthy House* book.[1] Have you discussed with Barbara and Hilton any of the specified products noted in the book to check for sensitivity, and would any of the release agents seal the form boards from the harmful release agents that were used on the last job? I think we should have the specific product selected prior to the foundation contractor's final pricing as the contractor would always select the least expensive product for the job. If the product did seal the forms then I would also not have to enquire about the use of new forms and the expense that would ultimately be passed on to the customers.

Geoff replied:

> I think we should get a form board from one of your foundation contractors and seal it with 'AFM Hard Seal'. I realize it will be a challenge to get the board to accept the seal as it is probably already so saturated with other release agents, but I think it could be worth a shot. The idea being

that it will create a continuous seal and contain the other agents. From there we could test it with Barbara and if it seems fine, we could then add our vegetable oil or Bio-Form (or equivalent) release agents and test again.

The conversation brought up a lot of issues for Barbara, who replied:

I would prefer that we use *Prescriptions for a Healthy House* as our guide. It is written by people who are experts. Whenever I have chosen not to heed the advice of my environmental doctor because it didn't seem necessary, I've regretted it.

The *Healthy House* book says that the use of petroleum-based form oil as a release agent is prohibited. This is really clear language. They also offer four other alternatives. Who is able to explore the other four alternatives and let us know how available the materials are and the cost?

There are also suggestions for sealing concrete on page 78 of the *Healthy House* book. This seems like a good step to take to reduce possible mold or radon problems. Speaking of which, in the book it says that ideally concrete should cure for a minimum of 28 days. Is it possible to do this?

Also, who is checking on the concrete mix? There are also guidelines for this, such as no admixtures are to be used.

I am not sure who orders the materials for a project like this. I'm finding myself in a challenging position because I don't want to be overbearing. But I've also had the experience of not asking enough questions and suffering the consequences later.

Dyson Simpson, who was costing the construction for Wilson Project Management, responded:

First of all, we are relying on you to make these points and ask these questions. Out of all of us you know the most about healthy provisions. By the end of the project we will all be experts.

Jeff Pepper is looking after the details such as the concrete mix, sealers, etc. I assure you he is on it. With each component we will need to take what the book is telling us to do exactly, get a price to do it, compare it to the budget and either proceed or find acceptable alternatives that provide you the same comfort but are more affordable. Either way, the ball will be in your court to provide direction.

The budget is designed to handle this type of project. However, I am certain that there will be times that the book is not offering us a solution that is affordable. In this case we will all put our heads together and present to you possible solutions. At the end of the day the first priority is that this house works for you, period. The second priority is that we come in on budget. We will do everything we can to complete both. I hope this eases your concerns.

We have been in contact with EcoInhabit and they will be providing many products for the job and will offer consulting. I understand that you have some experience with them and I assume that you trust in their competency. <u>Perhaps it would be best if a local expert was found that we could include in on our discussions concerning affordable solutions.</u>[2]

...

Jeff is looking into the different options for materials for the concrete. The problem with the recommended release agents is the old agents are still on the form boards. So that is why Geoffrey made the suggestion he did with the Hard Seal. Then if we do that we can then use one of the recommended agents. The other option is to buy a new set of forms, which is costly.

Never hesitate to raise your concerns.

While we appreciated the reassurances from Wilson, the interchange left us uncertain about our ability to achieve a completely healthy outcome. We loved the design on paper. But the planned use of reinforced concrete in the exterior walls and slab, and the need for form boards and release agents in the construction process, raised a lot of questions about chemical off-gassing for us. Maybe we really did need an independent consultant on healthy building who could provide some answers.

We found Robert Stellar's office a half-flight of stairs below an eyewear store and a bead shop on a small side street in the town of Thornbury, an hour north of our site. Robert's expertise had been highly recommended by EcoInhabit, a local retailer of green products and a consultant to Wilson on our project. According to his website, he had impressive credentials: a certified Building Biology Environmental Consultant and Inspector, former director of the International Institute for Building-Biology® and Ecology, and a consultant on new home construction in Germany, Canada, the U.S., and Brazil. He seemed to be exactly the type of resource we needed.

Robert has a very quick mind and a serious, Germanic style. It didn't take him long to determine that we were novices, and he proceeded to navigate us through one of his hour-long PowerPoint presentations on the principles and tools of building biology.[3]

All very interesting and valuable material; we wished we had seen it a year earlier. But now we were well along in the process and feeling pushed to get our project on schedule. Could he take some time with the plans we had in hand and help us find healthy alternatives to concrete admixtures, contaminated form boards and toxic release agents?

What ensued over the next hour was a revelation to us. We learned about concepts like "breathing walls" and thermal masses, why and how we could eliminate drywall and vapor barriers, how electromagnetic fields are created and mitigated. We discussed the use of insulated blocks for the walls, the necessity of replacing steel rebar with fiberglass rebar, and the proper design and construction of windows. By the end of our time with Robert, it was clear to us that we would have to make major changes in materials to get the house we were learning we wanted, and even needed. Perhaps we wouldn't adopt all of the materials or processes Robert recommended but enough to ensure that we would get a truly healthy home. It would take time and it would probably cost more. But knowing what we now knew was possible, compromise seemed out of the question.

The next day we pulled together our notes in an email to Superkül and Wilson. In fairness to everyone, especially Robert, this was our interpretation of the information we had been given:

> We had a very productive two-hour meeting yesterday with Robert Stellar of Breathing Easy in Thornbury. We'll leave you to check out his website, www.breathing-easy.net, to get his credentials, but we can tell you that we were very impressed with the scope of his insight and ideas on creating a home that "doesn't make people sick." Following is a summary of his recommendations for our house, all of which he has personal experience with:
>
> • Use Durisol block for the exterior and interior walls. Suggest you Google "Durisol Canada" to check out the properties to this impressive material. Use "outsulation" for optimum heat retention (as is code in Germany). Parge the exterior for wind barrier (code) and finish with wood, stone or concrete.

- Create a breathing house by eliminating vapor barriers so that walls, floors and ceiling are diffusible and hygroscopic. Durisol block, especially if combined with a wall finish like American Clay, will both absorb and give off moisture. Building biologists call this the "third skin" approach.

- Create a thermal mass in the walls by incorporating hot water heating lines inside the Durisol block rather than in the floors. This creates an infrared effect that is more penetrating to the skin, more efficient and healthier than radiant floor heating.

- Install the electrical lines in conduit inside the Durisol block to minimize electromagnetic radiation [EMR]. We recognize there may be some issues about trades working together at this stage in the project but we're sure WPM [Wilson] can deal with this.

- Windows: ensure they have a metal vapor barrier, with aluminum exterior and wood interior structure.

- Don't use drywall if possible. We really like the finish of American Clay (americanclay.com), which can be applied directly to

Durisol block and would lend a very natural (and healthy) complement to the cedar ceilings. The clay is available from EcoInhabit.

- EMR issues: No steel rebar — only fiberglass rod in the Durisol block and slab. And no steel roof because of its propensity to create electromagnetic fields, echoing the comments of our consultant at the Environmental Health Center in Dallas.

- On spray foam insulation in general, his concern was not the main product, like soy, but the reactant.

Given the design and size of the house, it was Robert's opinion that these changes were relatively easy to incorporate. We really don't know, but we do know that we like the thinking behind his suggestions and his commitment to a healthy living environment.

We also imagine that you may find this kind of information, at this stage in the project, annoying or at least inconvenient. This is totally new to us, too. But we would like you to seriously consider adopting these ideas, and getting in touch with Robert, and to do it in the spirit of challenge and learning. We realize that it might cost us a little more, but having come into contact with this information we feel we can't settle for a more conventional approach (and we know you've pushed the envelope already). Let's push it a little more and see what we can create that's not only great design but also great living. Many thanks for considering all of this.

Whatever feelings of panic, frustration, or annoyance may have crept in at Superkül or Wilson as a result of this new information, we were never aware of it. We suspected their professionalism would keep them focused on getting the best possible outcome whatever we decided, but their equanimity seemed almost saintly under the circumstances. André D'Elia, the lead architect, summed up everyone's approach with his response: "We'll look into the points mentioned. We do have concerns with some of the recommendations — some will impact costs as well as the schedule."

It's necessary to say that, at this point in the design and tendering process, many of the major components of the proposed construction seemed to us relatively conventional for a healthy house. The back wall, which in the final design was doing partial duty as a retaining wall, was to be concrete reinforced with steel rebar. The same approach would be used for the two side walls as well as a massive wall holding back the hill looming over the northwest corner of the house. The roof material was specified as standing-seam steel. The interior finish, while adapted to minimize health impacts, was nevertheless fairly typical in its specifications: studs, vapor barrier, insulation, drywall and paint.

Stellar's suggestion of Durisol insulated forms for the walls was, to us, a stroke of genius. (I will have more to say about the product in the next lesson on materials.) What captured our imagination was Durisol's natural ingredients, high recycled content, and imperviousness to rot and mold. Because the blocks were insulated and then filled with concrete after they were laid, we could put natural clay right on top of the block, just like smooth plaster. That would eliminate in one stroke all the standard components of wall construction — vapor barrier, insulation,

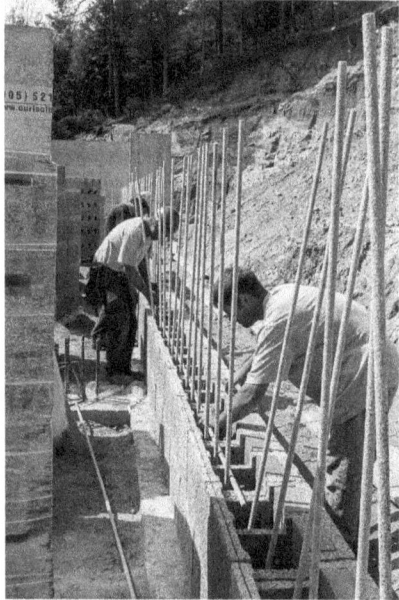

Tying-in the fiberglass rebar in the Durisol block. The cavity was filled with cement. Note the insulation on the outward-facing side of the block cavity.

drywall — and we would have perimeter walls that, for most of their extent, would be hygroscopic; in other words, capable of taking in and letting out water vapor in the form of humidity. It was the "breathing wall" idea, and it captivated us. A few days later, the structural engineers gave the block walls and fiberglass rebar their blessing and sent us another bill.

We were also fascinated by Stellar's idea of creating a thermal mass by incorporating the hot water lines in the Durisol block rather than in the floors. The idea is to create an infrared effect that is more penetrating to the skin, and more efficient and apparently healthier than in-floor heating. André's opinion was:

> This may not be practical in this case. The north wall has millwork along it and a portion of it makes up the north wall of the utility room. Thermal mass walls work better when the walls are unencumbered. The proposed in-floor radiant heating system is simply for floor warming — it doesn't really add to the heating of the space — it is primarily meant to take the chill off the floor. Where the in-floor warming really benefits the house is along the south glazing line — here the tubes are spaced closer together and create a

warm radiant curtain along the glass, hence reduce the heating load requirements of the furnace. A thermal wall along the north won't do this — we want the heating and warming to be where there is the greatest heat loss — by the windows.

Superkül didn't recommend that the interior walls be constructed of Durisol block because of coordination issues with plumbing, electrical and other services. They proposed, and we ultimately built, wood stud walls with paperless wallboard and American Clay.

A couple of months prior to these extensive changes, we had taken an earlier iteration of the plans to Carolyn Gorman at the Environmental Health Center in Dallas. She was acquainted with the authors of *Prescriptions for a Healthy House* and been a great resource to us on previous house renovations. Of the many recommendations she made, one of the most interesting was to keep any electrical wiring at least eighteen inches below the proposed steel roof. We wondered why. It was so that the electrical field surrounding the wiring wouldn't latch on to the broad conductive surface of the steel roof, creating a much larger electric field and with it the risk of significant health effects over time. This was the same reason why Robert Stellar recommended rethinking the steel roof as well as switching from steel to fiberglass reinforcing rod in the perimeter walls. Fiberglass, in contrast to steel, has low electrical conductivity and is electromagnetically neutral.

Very early on, Marianne, our consulting architect, had asked if we would consider a green roof. Now, with a simpler design and a stronger imperative, a green roof seemed like a good, if more costly, solution. Its three layers of membranes and a growing medium over plywood decking would eliminate steel in the roof over the living area, except for two steel support beams, which could be grounded. And it would give us more flexibility for recessed ceiling lighting. André sent us an email: "Judging from the photos Geoff took today [at his site visit], with all the vegetation on the hill, a green roof would look amazing and really blend into the hill and landscape." We took a deep breath and told them to get a quote.

It seemed like we were on our way to an even better house than we had expected. Yet the new direction the construction was taking as a result of our questioning set in motion a variety of unintended consequences. None were insurmountable, but each challenged the team's knowledge, experience with materials, and reliance on trusted suppliers and trades. And, of course, the schedule. All of this was ultimately our responsibility as owners who had questioned the status quo. But behind the scenes, it caused a flurry of cascading effects of which, at the time, we were unaware.

Jeff Pepper was doing his best to keep to the original budget. "Even $5,000 was a big issue," he recalled, "so being uncomfortable was having to call the rep from Durisol knowing it's the only product we can use and they're the only ones capable of supplying it. And there aren't a lot of people who lay Durisol blocks, so they're price setters — you basically pay what their price is. We knew that would impact the cost."

Time and cost issues were also exacerbated by the structural engineers' amendment to the plans. With the foundation and lower part of the back wall of the house now doing double duty as a retaining wall, Durisol's standard twelve-inch block wasn't up to the job. Our project required a fourteen-inch insulated block, a special order requiring weeks for custom production.

Sourcing fiberglass rebar was even more challenging for Superkül and Wilson. The product is typically used in large commercial projects like bridge decks, nuclear plants, and electric smelters. Suppliers are geared for commercial-size orders, not a small application with custom requirements like ours. "Like Durisol, there was only one manufacturer we could work with who would sell us the size and amount we needed," Jeff Pepper told me. "If it was steel rebar, we could have had twenty-foot lengths on site the next morning; we'd have gotten some benders and bent it to our needs. You can't just bend fiberglass. All those corners needed to be manufactured to the engineers' specs, and that was a two-week wait until they could get our order done."

We were now becoming resigned to the likelihood that we would not have a finished house by our goal of the following summer. Skids of Durisol block and fiberglass rebar were eventually delivered to the site as promised, but the project was far behind where we, probably unreasonably, felt it should have been by this time. Then the installation of the Durisol proceeded more slowly than we imagined it would. We were very aware that none of this would have been an issue for standard reinforced concrete walls. But +*House* was shrugging off the standard and embracing the prototype, even for a healthy house. We had asked our questions and were now living out the frustrating implications of the answers.

Construction proceeded, more or less conventionally, throughout the fall. The Durisol foundation rose nearly seven feet from the footings and was backfilled with soil from the site and topped off with aggregate in preparation for the hydronic heating lines and concrete slab. The front and back grades were established, and the crew returned to install the above-grade Durisol walls. The carpenters moved in to frame and clad the roof and, just before the first major snow, closed in the front window wall with plywood so Jeff could get the heaters on. We were relieved. Work could continue through the winter.

Our email questioning the use of chemical release agents on concrete form boards had led to dramatic changes in the major materials used in the house. But that email also posed a question that had gone unanswered: "Who is checking on the concrete mix?" With the pouring of the concrete slab scheduled for mid-December, the important question of the concrete, how it is finished and with what materials moved to the center of everyone's attention.

The authors of *Prescriptions for a Healthy House* were quite clear on the issue. To paraphrase their recommendations, the concrete should have "only clean, natural mineral aggregates" — no recycled materials or fly ash. Further, "no admixtures should be used." This eliminated retarders, accelerators and plasticizers—compounds that alter the setting time of concrete or the ratio of water to cement — that often contain potentially harmful ingredients. The concrete installer assured us by email that he had talked to Lafarge Ready Mix, the concrete supplier: there would be no recycled materials in the concrete.

"Fly ash," he said, "is the only material that is a by-product that isn't natural." Could it be tested for heavy metals or other toxic substances, we asked? Our research showed that most fly ash used as a concrete additive was a by-product from coal combustion and, despite some 'green' advantages like recycling, was a possible source of heavy metal contamination.

Superkül worked with engineers at Lafarge and the Ready Mixed Concrete Association of Ontario to find a solution to our concerns. By early December, we received a letter from Lafarge with their assurance:

> The concrete mix designed for the project... does not contain any supplementary cementing materials such as slag or fly ash. Also this product does not contain any chloride accelerators. The mix to be used is 25MPa non-air 10mm (3/8") stone. The mix code is RMXUH25N2MX.

Unknown to Wilson or the concrete installer, however, Lafarge had added extra Portland cement to make up for the volume of additives it would normally have used in its mix. The slab cured far more quickly — and far harder — than usual. That made the cutting of expansion joints to prevent the concrete from cracking not only extremely difficult but also prone to chipping. All of that had to be painstakingly repaired before the house was finished.

More concerning still was our search for a concrete "densifier" and sealant. A densifier aids in the hardening of the concrete surface during the diamond grinding process needed to smooth out imperfections from the pour and troweling. A sealant does just as it sounds — protects the concrete surface from being stained by spills. We plowed through manufacturers' websites in search of their products' ingredients, Material Safety Data Sheets (MSDS), and environmental claims. The chemistry was overwhelming, the MSDSs inconclusive or non-existent, and the claims varied wildly by product and manufacturer. It was very concerning: the concrete was a major element of the interior of the house and completely exposed throughout most of it. Barbara's frustration with getting the right information to ensure her health would be protected is evident in an email she sent just before Christmas, 2010:

This is a real challenge from a health perspective. I found one densifier that claims to be VOC compliant, but its MSDS says that in high concentrations it can cause headache, nausea, respiratory tract irritation, and so on. I also looked at *Xtreme Hard Densifier* and *Hermetix* densifier and both contain nanoparticles. Neither company provides MSDSs despite claims of no VOCs and no odor.

I'm appending the conclusion of a 2008 study done by scientists in Quebec about the potential effects of exposure to nano particles. Exposure to the particles is the key question. What protective gear are the concrete people required to use and why? Are nanoparticles sealed in after the grinding is finished and the product hardens on the floor? Can anyone really answer that question because there's been scientific testing? If not, can they be sealed in (to the extent we know if nano-level particles can be glued down)? What's the potential exposure to nanoparticles from normal wear and tear, because long-term or concentrated exposure is clearly not good.

I have to say that I feel very uncomfortable about any of the products that I've researched so far.

We never did settle on the supposedly essential densifier. The diamond grinding went ahead without one and to good effect: we have a polished concrete floor with great character. Better still, we have fewer potentially harmful chemicals to worry about. We didn't have the same option of simply eliminating a sealant. While we were trying to find the least-bad option — we eventually found a good choice — Jeff had to get on with the project:

> The sealer for the concrete was a complete nightmare. We couldn't pick a sealer but we had to go on with the construction, so I had to cover the floors. If anyone had dropped a coffee, we would have wrecked the floors, and we would have had to chip it out. That was terrifying. I don't know how many sealers we looked at, but it was all volatile, horrible stuff. By the time you moved in, it probably would have been inert, but we weren't willing to take that chance.

If you have experience in construction, some — perhaps much — of our questioning might appear amateurish. We were aware of that possibility. We didn't do it to be contrary or vexing or pseudo-professional. We questioned because we had to advocate for ourselves. It was our responsibility to express our wishes and concerns because not to do so would have left us open to someone else's interpretation of our needs. Considering the natural inclination of trades to use whatever materials they consider best for their business — faster, cheaper, better, proven — the odds were not in our favor that they would be thinking about healthy indoor environmental quality. We might get lucky, but given the many thousands of chemicals and compounds that remain untested for their impact on air quality and human health, it was most likely we would not.

Seeking answers along with the experts, and questioning until we were satisfied with the answers, was one of the best lessons we learned in building +*House*. It did lead us through unexpected turns, added occasional frustration and some additional cost.[4] But it did lead to a far healthier outcome for us and valuable learning for most everyone involved.

Notes

1   *Prescriptions for a Healthy House*, 3rd Edition, known to the team as "The Book."
2   Dyson's emphasis.
3   We've included the very useful 25 Principles of Building-Biology in the Appendix.
4   It's important to say that, apart from changes we approved to the scope of the project to achieve a better outcome, Wilson Project Management, thanks to the oversight of Jeff Pepper, brought the project in on budget. It wasn't an easy job.

Lesson 5:

It's (Mostly)
About the Materials

Early in the design stage of *+House*, on a cold, gray afternoon in late January 2010, Barbara and I were holed up in a downtown Toronto hotel room waiting for a visit from Superkül. We had traveled from Dallas specifically for this meeting, which would be our chance to interview two contractors vying for the opportunity to build our home. But the meeting also began a strange ritual that would continue throughout the project.

One of the challenges in building a healthy home is identifying the specific materials that will "work" for the people who will live there — in other words, materials that will not make them sick and, ideally, contribute to improving health. We knew that *Prescriptions for a Healthy House* identified a great variety of materials, from concrete to paint, that could help create a healthy living environment. Were newer or better materials now available? And what would work — or not work — for

Barbara's specific sensitivities? Apart from the obviously toxic products, like those containing volatile organic compounds (VOCs), we really didn't know.

That put the onus of initial product research squarely on Superkül's shoulders. "We always wanted more than one product," recalled André D'Elia, "in case that product didn't work. In fact, we wanted at least three. If all three failed, then we'd be stuck, and that's why we did more than what *Prescriptions* specified. We used the book like we use the building code. We'd refer to it as our first step, then go after alternatives — local, more or less recycled content, that sort of thing."

From Geoff Moote's perspective — Geoff was the project architect driving the details — a lot of architects will look at new materials that are interesting or trendy. Designing a healthy house required evaluating materials in a different way. We needed to know whether they off-gas toxic fumes like formaldehyde. What were their performance characteristics compared to standard products? What kind of reaction could they cause when used in conjunction with other products?

"Some of the products we didn't like at all, and some were really interesting," Geoff told us. "We never would have found them if we hadn't done this project. Even for something as simple as the substrate for the millwork, I must have spoken to 40 or 50 different suppliers across Canada and the U.S. to find an acceptable board. Overall, I'd say the house was 65 percent new product for us. It was a lot of up-front research. That was really the defining difference."

We gave Superkül a soft mandate to "think green." We wanted them to consider using recycled content if it would not detract from the air quality in the house, and here we occasionally found a dissonance. The idea of sustainability that underlies recycled content is fundamentally about reducing or conserving resources, whether energy or materials. But building healthy is first and foremost an intention about the occupant. Will the built space support health and well-being now and into the future?

Products manufactured from recycled materials, while a smart use of what would once have been considered waste, may not work for the immune-compromised person who must live with them. Many of these nominally green products can contain irritants such as formaldehyde-based glues. And the recycled content may also hold trace amounts of potentially harmful chemicals involved in the original manufacturing process. It was a lesson Superkül learned early on while testing products with Barbara — recycled did not automatically equate with healthy, at least for her.

Product performance was also an issue. While there are apparently green or healthy equivalents to products that are the industry standard, the team didn't feel confident that they could meet the challenge of issues like waterproofing against the steep hill on our site. There were 'peel and stick' products that didn't stick, and there were others that simply didn't have the specifications to stand up to the challenge. That left us with proven products like Blue Skin waterproofing. It was unlikely that they would test well with Barbara, but they would have to be used in the construction. We were fine with outside use only, at least conceptually. We didn't really know what would work.

We opened the hotel room door to find André and Geoff each pushing a luggage cart piled high with cartons. Inside the boxes were hundreds of sample products that might be used in the construction of *+House*. Superkül had obviously done their research. Now it was up to Barbara to identify those products she could not tolerate as well as those she could.

So began the ritual of smelling almost every product that went into the construction, from corten steel to curtain tracks. André handed Barbara the proposed product, and she inhaled and waited for the reaction while Geoff took notes on her reported reactions. A few examples from his notes:

Material	Result	Notes / Observations
Concrete floor, epoxy finish	Concern	Small reaction, further research required into concrete sealant by AFM Safecoat
Cold rolled steel, black patina	Concern	Detectable odor
Douglas fir, solid sawn	Good	Very comfortable with material
MDF (Arreis)	Concern	Odor from adhesive, could test with AFM
Rigid polystyrene insulation	Concern	Caused discomfort, exterior or encased may be acceptable
Window sample, oak & teak	No good	Fresh sample, no time to off-gas, will experiment with AFM, wood species OK
Corian	No good	Caused general discomfort

It is possible that the hotel room environment itself could have been an issue for Barbara, but we had stayed at that hotel before without much of a problem. For some severely compromised people, though, it might not work at all. Finding a relatively neutral space is important to the success of the sniff-testing process, as is taking a baseline 'measurement' of your level of reactivity before the testing begins.

There's no question that sniff-testing is very subjective, and Barbara does not in general recommend it. But it's expedient compared to a more scientific approach.

More rigor would have required the preparation and injection of hundreds of antigens made from potential building products, like the process that Barbara went through to gauge her sensitivity to foods, grasses, trees and so on at the Environmental Health Center. The human sense of smell is highly evolved, and chemical compounds in the form of smells go directly to the brain via the olfactory nerve. Barbara wasn't trying to identify smells, however. She was gauging her reaction to the chemicals that were inherent in the products, whether that be headache, agitation, tiredness, sneezing, even a sense of disorientation — of feeling "spacey," as she described it. Through the course of several hours of sniffing construction materials, she experienced all of these, headache being her predominant reaction to the products. By the end of the afternoon, she was feeling nauseous, disoriented, and overwhelmed from the chemical load, and it was several more days until she felt relatively well again.

Meanwhile, Superkül had their own uncertainties with the testing. According to André, "the main thing we were concerned with were the things you don't see. We really wanted to make sure those individual products worked. Then, if they were fine individually, how would they work with a collection of other materials coming together? That was the big unknown for us — the additive effect. We kept saying, 'it may be fine now, but what happens when you pair it with a few other things?' We were pretty confident that if one product tested fine on its own and another tested fine as well, the likelihood of an adverse reaction was probably small. But there's no way to test interactions without actually building the house or doing a one-to-one mockup. You just don't know."

Even before the testing phase, Superkül rejected dozens of potential construction components they knew would not react well with Barbara, a process they later claimed taught them as much about healthy building as the products they eventually specified for *+House*. In the end, only a few products used in the construction didn't test well with Barbara, and most of those were on the exterior or isolated in one way or another from the living space. Where we could not avoid a material that off-gassed — even a natural off-gassing like the cedar ceiling — we treated it with an AFM Safecoat product (we used several of their products in the project) that worked well for us in previous renovations.

"The Safecoat products were our fallback," Geoff said. "We knew that if something didn't test well at first, but then tested well with the sealant, we'd be okay. The windows were a good example. The wood on the windows was fine, but it has to be treated to stand up to weather. Since the standard sealant is usually the problem in terms of off-gassing, we specified the Safecoat product. The big challenge was getting the window manufacturer to buy into that, because he had his own processes and preferences. He would come back with other suggestions that we knew wouldn't work. But he used the Safecoat sealant, reluctantly and with a few application problems, and eventually he was very happy with the result."

The list below is the final list of major materials for *+House*. A word of caution, however: the products we used were the ones that worked for us. Your specific sensitivities or health concerns should guide your final selection.

Major As-Built Products and Components

- Concrete footings & retaining wall, fiberglass re-inforcing throughout. No ad-mixtures (e.g., fly ash, accelerators) in the concrete floor mix.

- **Durisol** recycled wood ICF block. Ad-mixture free concrete, Rockwool insulation and fiberglass rein-forcing in the cavity.

- **Rub 'r Wall** fluid applied damp-proofing, rear wall and foundation walls.

- Exposed concrete floors (except in master bath: por-celain tile), no ad-mixture. **Eco-Etch Pro** and **Acri-Soy** clear satin sealant.

- Glulam Douglas fir beams and columns at south wall (urea-formaldehyde free glue). Laminated veneer lumber (LVL) & FSC-Certified framing lumber (kiln dried) as secondary framing.

- **DensArmor Plus** paperless wallboard for interior walls.

- Interior walls finished with **American Clay** natural earth plasters. Loma base coats and Porcelina finish coat.

- **BASF WallTite** polyurethane spray insulation on ceiling (zero VOC).

- Rigid polystyrene insulation used only above the roof sheathing, outside only.

- Painted metal corrugated roofing on overhangs of house, and on garage.

- **Xero-Flor** green roof system above the living area of the house.

- Clear cedar tongue and groove cladding throughout, left unfinished. Clear cedar also used on interior ceiling, finished with **AFM Safecoat Acrylaq** satin sealant. Cedar roof fascia throughout.

- Windows and doors are oak interior with teak exterior. Oak finished with gloss AFM Safecoat Acrylaq sealant, exterior left unfinished. Fabricated by Radiant City. **Eco Insulated Glass** used throughout.

- Medium gauge corten steel used at sill of lift/slide doors on south walls, and bottom trim around perimeter of house at base of cladding.

- **Stuv** high efficiency fireplace, with cold-rolled steel surround. Steel mantle finished with a matte black **AFM** paint. Through-porcelain tile on hearth, **Progetto Pavimenti** tile.

- Through-porcelain tile on bathroom walls, master bathroom floor, no glaze. **Progetto Pavimenti: Bianco m.**

- Millwork of rift-cut white oak veneer plywood without urea-formaldehyde, using water-based glue. Sealed with **Valspar** and top coat of **AFM Safecoat.**

- **Icestone** counter tops (recycled glass with concrete) throughout, sealed with **Protex by Tenex.**

- **Shearweave** Non-PVC roller shades, by **Solarfective.**

- Drapes of 80% hemp / 20% silk fabric by **Effort Industries (**product #10125). Regular cotton blend lining —PC Sateen Plus, col: ivory, 50% cotton, 50% polyester. Blackout lining for bedroom areas — Thermo Soft Blackout, col: ivory, 65% polyester, 35% cotton.

- **Artemide Surf 300** Halogen wall light along south beam. **Iris Halo Eyeball** recessed downlights in ceiling. **FLOS KAP** pendant lights above kitchen island. **Artemide Dioscuri** wall light above vanities. **Tolomeo** reading lamps in master bedroom. **FLOS Glo-Ball** above dining table

- **Lutron Diva** switches and dimmers

This list of 'as-built' materials, together with the very broad range of product suggestions in *Prescriptions for a Healthy House*, should provide a good starting point for determining which products may work for your home construction or renovation. A more comprehensive listing of less-toxic options is available on the Healthy Building Network's Pharos Project.[1] Now in its third version, this excellent subscription site currently evaluates some 1,600 building products from 300 manufacturers and profiles 37,500 chemicals and materials for their health and environmental impacts.

The balance of this chapter focuses on the major components used in the construction of *+House*. We discussed concrete in the last chapter. What follows are some thoughts on the lessons we learned from, and about, Durisol block and American Clay, as well as the custom millwork that is a major feature of the house.

Durisol

The original specification for the north, east and west exterior walls of +*House* called for fairly standard house construction — a combination of reinforced concrete or stud walls with insulation, vapor barrier and gypsum drywall. These were to be built on a foundation of reinforced concrete and slab-on-grade. As I related earlier, our meeting with Robert Stellar, a Certified Building Biology Environmental Consultant and consultant on healthy home construction, changed all of that, with the exception of the concrete floor.

The changes grew out of the first of two hours we spent with Stellar learning about the principles of "baubiologie" or building biology. It was a completely new concept to us. The ideas originated in Germany in response to a variety of problems with post-war housing construction. The ideas were then brought to North America in 1987 when acclaimed architect Helmut Ziehe founded the International Institute for Building-Biology and Ecology, now located in Santa Fe, New Mexico. Stellar is a former director of the Institute.

The Institute's mission is to help communities and individuals create healthy homes, schools and workplaces — environments that are free of pollutants from the air, water, and electromagnetic spectrum. Or as we like to think of them, environments that support the well-being of their occupants.

Our sense was that the touchstone of the building biology discipline is its "25 Principles of Bau-Biologie," which I have reproduced in the Appendix. Taken in totality, these principles and the conditions of construction they stipulate seem utopian. But individually they made a great deal of sense, especially to neophytes like us who were simply committed to building as healthy a house as possible. There were a handful of these principles — their place in the list of 25 is in brackets — that we recall Stellar emphasizing as he reviewed the proposed working drawings for our house:

- Use natural and unadulterated building materials. (5)

- Use wall, floor, and ceiling materials that allow air diffusion and are hygroscopic. (6)

- Indoor air humidity shall be regulated naturally. (7)

- An appropriate balance of thermal insulation and heat retention is needed. (9)

- The air and surface temperatures of a given room need to be optimized. (10)

- Eliminate or reduce man-made electromagnetic radiation as much as possible. (19)

Not surprisingly, Robert had an opinion about the type of building materials that could meet such a broad-based mandate. He strongly recommended Durisol insulated concrete forms with fiberglass rebar. We had not heard of either.

Durisol blocks (**durisolbuild.com**), manufactured in Hamilton, Ontario, seemed to be an almost perfect product for many of the dictates of building biology. The insulated concrete forms (ICFs) are made from recycled softwood lumber waste that is chipped and then bonded with Portland cement. Moisture-resistant mineral fiber, known as rockwool, inside a portion of the cavity provides up to R-21 insulation value. Placed on the outer side of the hollow core of the block, this 'out-sulation' cannot sag over time like conventional insulation bats because the rest of the cavity is filled with reinforced concrete. Durisol blocks are also porous, durable, do not rot or decay and are impervious to vermin, termites and insects. Because of their high alkalinity, they do not support mold growth. And since they are manufactured from completely natural ingredients — no post-consumer or demolition waste is added — the forms don't contain or emit any toxic elements.

Our 'aha' moment came when Robert talked about the potential for the product to improve the air quality of the house. The Durisol material is hygroscopic, he explained, which means it can store and release moisture in the form of water vapor as required. Because it's permeable, it doesn't act as a vapor barrier like the plastic sheeting found in standard wall systems; it is more of a vapor regulator that helps keep relative humidity of the indoor air at healthy levels. We knew that was also another critical factor in eliminating the potential for mold growth.

We were converted. Stellar then went on to describe the benefits of using the Durisol walls to create a thermal mass. The walls are designed to literally absorb and give off heat or cooling over long periods of time, much like large rocks that absorb the energy of the summer sun will quickly melt the first snows of the winter with their stored heat. This could be enhanced, he said, by incorporating the hot water lines designed to warm the concrete floor directly into the walls. This would create an infrared effect that is more penetrating to the skin, and more efficient, and apparently healthier, than in-floor heating.

We ticked off all the building biology imperatives this approach would accomplish and sent Superkül and Wilson Project Management the evangelical email reproduced in the last lesson. As it transpired, Durisol would be a primary building product in *+House*, though not quite the way Robert Stellar envisioned.

We subsequently asked André how using Durisol ICFs affected Superkül's design, if at all: "It was the right house for Durisol because the house is rectilinear and fairly simple, with a back wall and two side walls. If it was more complicated, if the house was a different form, like two stories, it wouldn't be the right product. We would have used something else. Even the two windows on the west and east sides are punch windows. We made sure it was going to be very simple. It's the nature of the material, really. The blocks are big and funky, and it's hard to get them straight and true. You have to give a lot of tolerance."

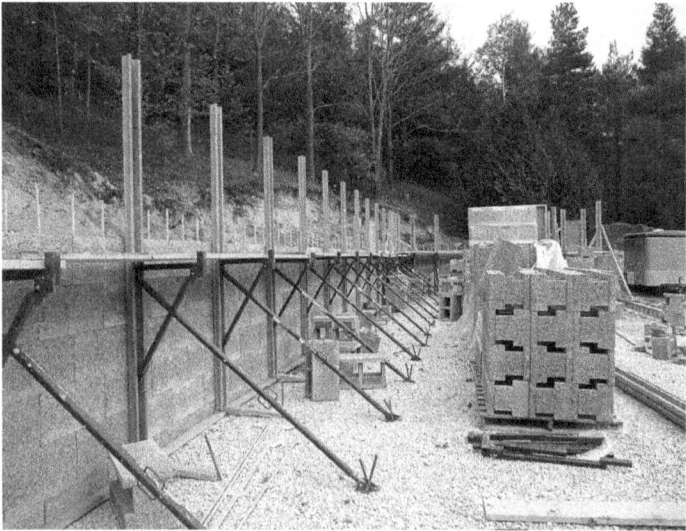

The Durisol block required constant alignment during construction to maintain the tolerance of the design.

We learned from Tim Singbeil, whose team at Dasein Construction installed the Durisol for *+House*, that tolerance — physical and psychological — is one of the reasons we don't see the product used in the construction of more North American buildings. The ICF manufacturing process causes slight variations in shape that make it more difficult and time-consuming for trades to install. A three-day process may stretch into a couple of weeks. Builders, especially production builders, don't want the added cost or grumbling trades, whatever the eventual health benefits for the occupants.

As Jeff Pepper, our site supervisor, viewed the challenge, "it isn't like a concrete block, where you can lay it perfectly straight and put a level on it. Durisol blocks aren't perfectly consistent, and they're dry stacked. When we filled the cavities with concrete as we went up, it would start to "snake" from the weight of the upper block. So Tim's crew would have to go back again and realign. And by the time we got up to 14 feet at the [front] corners, there was a lot of extra framing involved to keep the lines straight."

Among his many construction skills, Tim Singbeil is an expert in the residential and commercial use of Durisol block and has created a certification course for Durisol that is now required of builders who want to use the product. According to Tim, it was a difficult project, even for an experienced installer: "It's a contemporary house, so Jeff was after really high tolerances — within an eighth of an inch over about 90 feet. In some cases we were dealing with blocks that were a quarter inch out of square, in whatever direction you want to measure. We would push the imperfections to the outside wall, where they could be cleaned up in the strapping and siding process, and we were constantly adjusting for level and alignment. It certainly brought our game up a notch."

There was a lot of block to install. From the footings, the foundation walls, also made of Durisol ICFs, rose nearly seven feet. Because the foundation was to be back-filled for the slab, precise tolerances weren't as important there. The above-grade walls, however, had to be as close to perfectly even as possible. The finished interior would be clay applied directly on top of the Durisol, leaving the team with no chance to hide misaligned blocks behind conventional drywall. (That said, Durisol's composition of wood chips and cement enabled small variations on the inside walls to be leveled before the application of the clay.)

With the inherent variations in the blocks now on the outside of the walls, the foundation and rear wall demanded a waterproofing membrane that could accom-modate the unevenness of the block. Superkül specified Rub-R-Wall (**advancedcoatings.on.ca**), an innovative impermeable membrane that is spray-applied. One of

Rub-R-Wall's qualities is elasticity of up to 1800 percent, which enabled it to adapt to the wall's imperfections. It was an ideal product for our combination of no-fail waterproofing and the variations in the block. Above grade, the walls were a little less high-tech: standard wrap, then strapped and clad with tongue and groove clear cedar. The house wrap is an air barrier but not a vapor barrier, so it does not affect the breathability of the Durisol.

American Clay

To say that we were enthusiastic when we discovered American Clay at EcoInhabit is a significant understatement. Here was a product that singlehandedly accomplished some of our most deeply held goals for the house. Its blend of aggregates, clays and pigments didn't off-gas at all. Test results showed that the porous clay plaster finish would not support mold growth. Because it was porous, it could help regulate humidity by 'breathing' water vapor in and out, making the house more comfortable. And American Clay was exceptionally friendly environmentally, with nearly three-quarters of its volume coming from clean post-industrial recycled content.

'Green' and healthy were great, necessary in fact, but we also had aesthetic aspirations. We were taken by the quality of light that we saw reflecting off the samples at EcoInhabit. American Clay crushes post-industrial rock and shell waste into sand that forms the base of its "earth plasters." We didn't know why, but the product seemed to have a subtle reflectivity that made it feel vibrant and soft at the same time. We had certainly never seen a paint finish with remotely the same qualities.

We knew we wanted a product like this in the house, but, at this point in the process, Superkül was still specifying fairly standard interior walls finished with Safecoat paint. When Robert Stellar recommended Durisol blocks, he also made a strong case for using American Clay throughout the interior to enhance the 'breathing wall' qualities of the block. With the right clay composition, the product could be applied thickly like interior stucco or, in our case, like a smooth plaster, called porcelina. Fortunately, that approach made a lot of sense to Superkül as well.

The installation of the clay, however, was not as straightforward as drywall and paint. We contracted with specialist installers of the product for just the final finish coat, and our budget wouldn't allow a drywall and taping contractor as well as an expert in American Clay application. Wilson asked our drywall contractor — one of the best in Toronto — if they were up to the challenge of using an unfamiliar product. They were: how much different from typical drywall compound could a final coat of clay be? In fact, there was a big difference. "We still had a lot of work to install and tape the paperless drywall,[2] level and straighten the Durisol block areas," Jeff Pepper told us. "We also had to prepare all of the walls with a special wall primer mixed with American Clay sand for proper adhesion of the two final clay coats. Our tapers did get the walls perfectly leveled, primed and the base layer of clay on, but they were having a difficult time applying the second coat over the large wall areas. They were actually burning the finish, which we learned later was caused by our North American drywall trowels. Apparently the best application tools were handmade plaster trowels from Japan.[3]

"We had to bring in a specialist installer of American Clay from Toronto who had trained in France. He taught the tapers how to apply the final clay coat, leaving them with the smaller, more-manageable walls while the experts worked on the large surfaces. The challenge was getting the right compression of the final finish. Everyone could do it on the smaller areas but only he could compress consistently over a large area. With training from the experts and an investment in Japanese trowels, our tapers eventually got very good results, almost as good as the specialist."

American Clay, as we have discovered, is a strong and durable product. But it has other compelling qualities that we could not sense from simply looking at a small sample at EcoInhabit. Across a broad area, or throughout an entire house in our case, the clay lends a softness to the living space — a tangible "feeling on the back of the neck," as one visitor said. Even the more hard-edged qualities of contemporary design and furniture give way to a sense of comfort. Sitting in the completed house for the first time, André told us that "American Clay is a healthy product that really adds to the character of the space. Everything feels soft, like it absorbs the light. Edges kind of get smoother. It feels relaxing. Even the photos kind of capture that, a kind of haze. It's really refreshing."

And, as we experience it, regenerating.

Millwork

Of all the challenges we had in finding materials that would agree with Barbara, none tested our resolve to build healthy as the products that went into the cabinetry. The millwork in +*House* is a major functional component of every room. Our feeling was that the extensive use of built-in cabinetry was mandated by contemporary design — keep the lines simple and the surfaces uncluttered. Superkül agreed, but insisted on a more practical purpose for our needs. Unlike standalone furniture that accumulates dust on and under its surfaces, closed cabinets would minimize dust collection and make the house easier to keep clean. The few horizontal millwork surfaces in the house would be easily reached for cleaning. All the other cabinetry not in the kitchen or bathrooms should extend from the floor to the ceiling or be incorporated into a wall. So, for both design and health reasons, it was important to get it right.

As the design began to take on its final shape, we met with Superkül and Andy Johnston, the manufacturer, to discuss a strategy for the millwork. From a healthy building perspective, the issue was the total composition of materials in the millwork — the core or substrate of the board, the veneer surfaces and the glue that held them together. Why not eliminate all that by using solid wood, we asked? Solid wood will shrink, crack and warp, they said, so it's not suitable for the large panels we needed. Add in the additional labor required for finishing and solid wood could double the cost of the millwork. We crossed that possibility off the list.

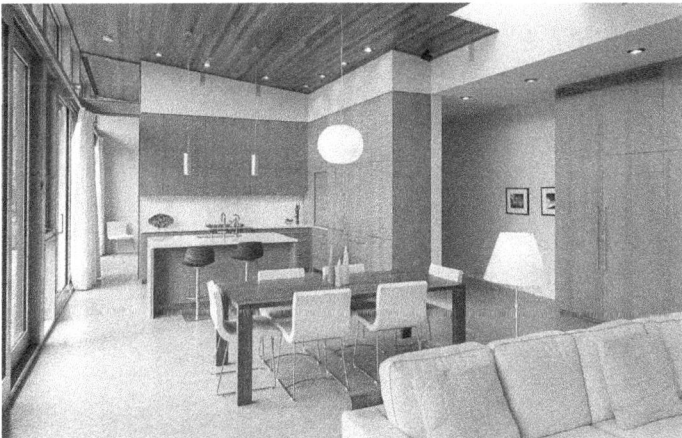

The millwork is a major design feature of the house – clean, functional and very attractive.

Geoff Moote of Superkül and Andy Johnston set out to find the best combination of components. While Geoff contacted manufacturers across North America, Andy was scouring the Internet. "Probably 95% of my research was on online," he said, "trying to find different articles, going through MSDS sheets from manufacturers, trying to make sense of what chemicals were in there to look for. Then I'd call and talk to tech people at the manufacturers or the sales people. I got some information from the *Healthy House* book. But typically they would direct me straight to straw board, which I'd heard was basically unusable because it doesn't bond together very well. So their suggestions weren't all that helpful.

"Most of my work was just combing through every piece of information I could find and try to make the best judgment from what I could learn. But I didn't find that there was a lot of clear, obvious help out there to direct me to what to use..."

In addition to the samples we had tested in our Toronto hotel room, we received regular shipments in Dallas that contained samples of combinations of substrates, glues, edge bands and veneers. Some were unsealed and others sealed once with Valspar and a second time with AFM Safecoat Hard Seal. Some had holes drilled through the veneer or no edge banding. Barbara would sniff-test each one and make notes on her reactions. They were never good. A typical report from her was, "we received the next shipment of cabinet samples this morning. Unfortunately, none of the samples were okay. I really reacted strongly to the glue and am still coughing. The sample that worked the best was the Sierra Pine until I smelled the edge, which is where I reacted to the glues. I did not react to any of the edge bands that were sent. I feel rather discouraged about all of this because I am cognizant of time and budget constraints. And I wish I wasn't quite so sensitive…

"Another important issue in regards to sealing seems to be holes in the board. If optional shelving holes are drilled into the boards then there is no sealant on the exposed holes. I reacted much more strongly to the boards that had holes drilled in them than to the ones that had been completely sealed. I'm sorry I don't have a different response for you."

And so it went in a dance of action and reaction, one partner not knowing how the other would lead or follow. Over several months, Barbara tested some 50 different combinations of materials, edging, finishes, and sealants for the millwork. Those samples represented a huge amount of research for Johnson and Superkül over the better part of two months. As Andy recalled, he had tried to be aware of the health issues of his work, but had never had to find the "right" product for a client with chemical sensitivities. His moment of illumination came when "I finally realized I wasn't looking for the perfect thing. I was looking for the acceptable thing." That threw the decision back on us to define acceptable. We didn't know a scientific method. Barbara would have to define it with her nose.

Non-formaldehyde panels like those from Uniboard, Panalam, Temple, Arreis, Encore and Purebond — some recommended in *Prescriptions for a Healthy House* — had tested too poorly with Barbara to be reconsidered. Andy felt he was out of options and the clock was running down. Once again, however, serendipity made an appearance in the form of an unscheduled visit by a sales rep for Hardwoods, a major North American supplier of sheet goods and lumber. He brought a sample of plywood Andy described as "amazing," though not for us. Further inquiry led us to Hardwoods' new "Dragon Ply" sheet in a version without formaldehyde, which was also manufactured in China under strict quality control. Barbara's reaction to an untreated sample was not perfect, but stayed within the bounds of acceptable. Though we were concerned about sourcing a key component of our healthy house from China, with just two months left before we intended to move into the house, we told Andy to order the plywood and get the cabinets into production.

Manufacturing and Installation. Before he began the manufacturing process, Johnston and his team went through "countless strategies" to avoid exposing the inside substrate. Because of Barbara's inconsistent reactions to combinations of woods and sealants, she and Andy had to work out a sealing strategy to prevent off-gassing. Andy preferred Valspar, a Green Guard-certified, no-formaldehyde lacquer that he had been using for years. Barbara wanted to use AFM Safecoat sealers, which we had used several times to good effect.

We reached a compromise. "We sealed everything — every surface of 105 sheets of plywood — with Valspar and then top-coated all that with the Safecoat," Andy said. "And wherever possible, we'd leave the panels in our spray booth, which is a large room with radiant heaters in it. We just cranked up the heat as high as possible and left the panels in there as long as we could. Barbara told us it would speed up the cure and off-gassing, and apparently it did."

There were other precautions as well. While cutting of the cabinet panels was completely standard, every edge had to have some sort of sealer on it, whether it be wood or liquid, to prevent the inevitable out-gassing. Each cabinet back, for example, which in normal manufacturing is simply screwed onto the cabinet box, had to be cut undersized to allow for a 1mm edge band. If a surface couldn't be banded, it was sealed with AFM Safecoat several times. Even the backs of cabinets, up against the wallboard, were treated with sealant. What's more, Johnson minimized the use of glues by screwing together the cabinets' biscuit joints wherever possible rather than using the standard 'belt and suspenders' approach of gluing *and* screwing the panels together.

The necessity of maintaining a consistent seal across all millwork surfaces also affected the team's thinking about installing the cabinetry. It became an issue of advance planning rather than on-site execution. Andy recalled that, "we were reluctant to scribe-fit anything, because if we had to shave anything down to make it fit the wall better that meant exposing the core of the plywood. So we really avoided that. In some ways it made our lives easier, and in other ways we had to make filler pieces better and more accurate so that they could be put into place. Anything that needed to be cut for some reason had to be coated with Safecoat. But we really did try to plan it so that we'd avoid that type of thing.

"There were a few pieces that we just ended up bringing back to the shop, re-edged them, re-sprayed them and then installed. Whereas if it had have been anyone else's house, we probably would have cut it off, sanded the edge and put it in and not worried about it. But as long as we knew this kind of thing in advance, we just planned for it."

I asked Andy if there was anything he learned on the project that surprised him. "The big realization," he said, "was that there's no real way to know what these allergic reactions are to, specifically. I thought it was cut and dried that most of these environmental allergies were to formaldehyde. I don't think that anymore. There are so many chemicals out there, and combinations of chemicals, that we don't know about."

Notes

1   **https://pharosproject.net**. According to the site, the Project: "evaluates 1,601 building products and components from 328 manufacturers, across 15 major product categories; the ingredients of 469 products are completely disclosed by 62 manufacturers; profiles 37,763 chemicals and materials for 25 health and environmental hazards, including carcinogenicity, mutagenicity, reproductive toxicity and endocrine disruption, against 62 authoritative lists of hazards issued by governments, NGOs and other expert bodies; rates 288 product certifications and standards and uses them in building product evaluations."

2   Superkül specified DensArmor Plus by Georgia-Pacific for the interior walls. According to the manufacturer's website, "DensArmor Plus® gypsum interior panels are ideal for moisture-prone commercial and residential interior spaces. This moisture-resistant wallboard incorporates fiberglass mats front and back, instead of paper facings, and a moisture-resistant core for superior moisture and mold resistance when compared to traditional paper-faced drywall."

3   Among the best are handmade trowels by Yamanishi. See **https://sites.google.com/site/japanesetrowels/yamanishi-trowels**. For a primer on Japanese plastering, see **http://japaneseplastering.com/japanese-trowels**.

Lesson 6:

Look for the Unseen

You will recall the story from the lesson "Know Yourself" about the property we were considering purchasing in Dallas where certain places in the house made Barbara feel "jittery." How even a skilled electrician couldn't account for the spikes in electromagnetic radiation and why, despite turning off the power at the main panel, relatively high levels of radiation persisted. It was a disturbing conundrum that made us withdraw our offer for a home we sincerely wanted.

Welcome to life in the field.

This book is not the place for a review of the extensive literature that catalogs how disruptive electromagnetic, radio, and microwave frequencies are to our bodies' functions, and particularly to those of young children. Suffice it to say that prolonged exposures, especially to radio and microwave frequencies emanating from devices such as cell phones, smart meters, and Wi-Fi, as well as from "dirty" electricity,[1] have been shown to affect the major electrical systems in the body: the brain (headaches, dizziness, insomnia, lack of focus, learning, and remembering); the heart (increase in arrhythmias); and the cells (increased long-term propensity to develop cancers[2]).

But let's face it: we're not going back to a hard-wired world. The Internet of (Interconnected) Things is upon us, and wireless is ubiquitous. The question is how to reduce our exposures. In finding answers to this question, we had a significant head start in designing and building *+House* — our location in the rolling hills of Mulmur.

Compared to the pervasive "electrosmog" of electromagnetic, radio frequency, and microwave pollution that now blankets urban, suburban, and even ex-urban environments, the site on which the house sits is positively pristine — a characteristic we didn't realize should be part of our original wish list, but ultimately one of the healthiest qualities of the home. The house is twenty minutes from the nearest town. It is shielded by the hill to the north from the closest cell tower and too far away from towers in other directions to register more than an occasional, faint signal. There are no major power lines, transformers, or industrial users in the vicinity. And we had the distinct advantage of working with new construction, which enabled us to minimize as many elements of electrosmog as we could.

So, how could we make the best of the good situation we had stumbled upon? Our vigilance against the unseen began, literally, at ground level.

Grounding. If not properly grounded, steel in homes can carry electrical currents that create EMF, and we had quite a bit of steel in the original design. That was the primary reason Robert Stellar, the building biologist we consulted, suggested that we switch from steel to fiberglass reinforcing bar in the foundation and above-ground walls, as well as in the slab. As we described in an earlier lesson, fiberglass rebar was difficult to get for a small project like ours but worth the logistical hassles because it does not conduct electrical or magnetic currents. Additionally, the electrical engineers and contractor assured us that all steel inside the living envelope such as beams, columns, and the fireplace surround could and would be grounded. Even large exterior elements like the rebar in the large exterior retaining wall and steel roof trim were grounded to minimize potential fields.

Roof. Both Carolyn Gorman of the Environmental Health Center and Robert Stellar were firmly against the original idea of a standing-seam steel roof. According to Gorman, unless wiring is at least eighteen inches below the steel, electromagnetic fields can form on the expansive conductive surface. The steel sheet can also reflect EMF and create "hot spots" in the home. We opted, at additional cost, for a green roof over the living envelope — several levels of non-metallic decking and membrane covered by a growing medium that supports small plants called cetums.

Electrical Panels. Our electrical engineers recommended placing the main panel in the garage, which is about ninety feet away from the house. The power lines from the main panel to the house travel in underground conduit and are distributed through a lower-voltage sub-panel located in the mechanical/laundry room inside the house.

A note on smart meters. *+House* has one, as required by our utility's terms of service, but it is installed on the wall of the garage, well away from where we spend our time. Smart meters use electronics rather than mechanisms to measure electricity consumption and time of use, which is intended to help utilities balance demand across the system. The meters need not be physically read each month because they transmit data over long distances by short-pulsed radio frequencies, just like a cell phone. And they transmit data literally thousands of times a day to a smart grid that links local areas and sends the information to the utility's computers for analysis and billing.

(How they do this at our home, where we can barely register a cell signal, is beyond my understanding.)

According to Health Canada, smart meters emit no more electromagnetic radiation than cell phones or Wi-Fi routers.[3] But as no long-term studies have been done on the effects of these devices — and the impact of these devices in aggregate in our living environments — that is a hotly contested assertion. "Smart Meters: Correcting the Gross Misinformation," written by a group of fifty scientists and public health professionals, lays out the concerns and argues strongly for reducing exposures to these pulsed radiations.[4] While our meter is well away from the house, we have nevertheless installed a stainless steel smart meter guard over the unit. The manufacturer claims the guard, which it sells online for $130.00, reduces radiation by as much as 99% without comprising the communications ability of the meter itself.[5]

Electrical Wiring. Wiring +*House* to ensure the lowest-possible level of electromagnetic pollution was an important issue for the architects and electrical engineers. The design minimized horizontal runs of wiring, which form a potential "girdle" of EMF around the living space, in favor of runs that began in the ceiling and terminated at plugs and switches throughout the space. It was not an easy task given the large, open plan of the house.

"The EMFs were a big challenge," said Geoff Moote, the project architect, during one of our debriefs. "Not conceptually, but you just don't know until you fire up the whole house." Several electrical contractors were scared away from bidding on the job because we had set a standard of less than one milliGauss on average throughout the living space. And, with a test before we moved in, the team would have to stand behind their work. "You gave me a Gaussmeter, but without the electricity hooked up, we didn't know," Jeff Pepper said with some exasperation. "But it was still my responsibility."

Superkül had originally specified that the wiring run through rigid conduit everywhere in the house. This type of conduit is expensive to install, with a lot of bending and junction boxes—not something our budget could accommodate. We told Jeff to do what he thought was right to reduce both the price and the EMF. The solution he developed with the electrician and Superkül was to use Romex non-metallic wire in BX flexible metal conduit throughout the living areas of the house. But it wasn't until the very end of the project, when all the connections had been made and all the three- and four-way switches were double-checked, that Jeff got a reading we were all happy with — an average of about 0.5 milliGauss.

It was that reading, especially at the head end of our bed, that helped us make the decision not to install what's known as a kill switch on the master bedroom circuits. Robert Stellar and others had advocated the use of such a switch, which cuts off the power to an individual circuit, on the circuit planned in the area of our bed. Simply flip on the switch before retiring — or when you're having a nap — and the sleep-disturbing electric fields associated with current flows are significantly reduced.

In the case of +*House*, the wiring in the vicinity of our bed was minimal: a reading lamp, plug and two switches on my side of the bed. Barbara's side of the bed has only a plug and hardwired reading lamp to avoid running wiring across the back of the headboard. We do not use a cordless phone or an electric clock radio. (In our Dallas home, where we did not have control of the wiring configuration, we installed and use a kill switch at night.) See *Prescriptions for a Healthy House* for an extensive discussion of the effects and mitigation of household electrical fields, as well as the use of kill and demand switches. You will find cost-effective solutions for both new and existing construction.

Lighting. One of several arenas in which sustainable living and healthy living clash is household lighting. In 2009, at the behest of the U.S. and Canadian governments, manufacturers announced that they would begin to phase out the production of standard incandescent light bulbs in 2012. Compact fluorescent bulbs (CFLs) were available that would work in the house but we didn't like the quality of light. Moreover, CFLs emit relatively high levels of radiofrequency and ultraviolet radiation that can migrate along the electrical circuit, which concerned us. Low-voltage halogen lighting necessitated mini-transformers to operate, a choice that would have amplified electromagnetic fields throughout the house. LED bulbs, while energy-efficient and less prone to high levels of EMF, were still very expensive at the time of construction. Our eventual choice was incandescent halogen floods, which are about thirty percent more efficient than standard incandescents and have a pleasing bright white color temperature. And yes, we did install high-quality dimmers, even though we knew they would emit some magnetic and RF fields when in use.

Internet and Telephone. One of the first questions we typically get from overnight guests is, "what's your Wi-Fi password?" And there's always that haven't-you-taken-this-healthy-thing-too-far look in their eyes when we explain that while we have Wi-Fi, we keep it turned off. And when we tell them there's no cell signal either, the looks can turn from a "really?" arch of the eyebrows to truly forlorn.

At the design stage of the project, we specified that the major rooms, our office and entertainment center be wired with ethernet cable to eliminate the possibility for radio frequencies on which Wi-Fi runs. It's not enough to leave the Wi-Fi radio on and connect the computer by ethernet. The radio needs to be turned off at the router. In our experience — we do this every night at our home in Dallas — the best way to do this so as to not 'confuse' the electronics is to access the router software via a browser window and change the configuration so the wireless is disabled. Most router instruction manuals will have details of this simple procedure.

Since our internet connection at +*House* is via a satellite link, as an additional precaution we placed the satellite dish on the hill above the garage. The modem is installed in the garage, well away from the house and in the winter months is kept warm by a single fluorescent bulb in a small plywood box. The cable to the router inside the house runs in the underground conduit along with the electrical feed and cable from the satellite television dish (also a good distance from the house).

We adopted the same strategy for our landline phones. Cordless phones, especially the newer digital models, can emit very high levels of radiofrequency pollution and EMF. The two office phones are hardwired, with corded handsets. And since our cell phones don't work at our location, we put them on airplane mode (so the batteries don't drain fruitlessly looking for a cell tower) and leave them out on the front hall, on the opposite side of the house from our bedroom. Just in case.

The Air We Breathe

We humans spend a lot of time indoors — as much as 90 percent according to Health Canada. Whether we're at home, driving our cars, taking public transportation, or working in offices or factories, the vast majority of our indoor time is spent in manufactured spaces built with materials that are predominantly synthetic or chemically processed. As discussed in an earlier chapter, these materials add to the increasingly heavy load of environmental toxins in our bodies, which a significant number of people have difficulty eliminating. And that can lead, as it did in Barbara's case, to allergic reactions or hyper-sensitivity to chemicals in the environment, both indoors and out.

During the design stage of +*House*, we worked out a three-part strategy with Superkül to ensure we would have the best possible indoor air quality: first, find as many materials as possible to which Barbara did not react; then seal-in the off-gassing of those materials we couldn't avoid; and, finally, keep the air fresh, filtered, and well-conditioned from season to season. As we neared the start of construction, we were very pleased with the care the team was taking with the sourcing and selection of materials. We felt that maybe a really healthy house was possible after all. And then we had another experience that drove home the importance of being vigilant about materials and the challenge of reducing the impact of chemical pollution when you don't pay enough attention.

Our plan during the summer of construction was to rent a house in Creemore, a village about a twenty-minute drive from the site. During our search for the property, we tried to give our real estate agent a good idea of the healthy house we intended to build. We trusted that she would have an understanding of what we needed in a rental house. And we were in Dallas by now, making trust an essential part of the transaction. The agent found a small bungalow that she believed would be ideal. It had been renovated the previous fall but, she assured us, would have six months to gas off. It looked fine from the pictures, though still obviously under construction when they were taken. We somewhat reluctantly signed the lease without an inspection.

As we discovered, we would have saved ourselves a huge amount of money, time and worry had we asked what should have been an obvious question: How does a newly renovated house in a cold climate passively off-gas during the winter? Not readily, nor naturally.

When I arrived on my own the following April to clear out our belongings from the old house on our property, the rental reeked with the chemical bouquet of conventional construction — drywall, paints, cabinetry, sealants. The renovation apparently completed the previous fall was not actually finished until December, and the house had, for the most part, been shut tight throughout the winter. I knew Barbara wouldn't be able to tolerate the brew of off-gasses that were sloshing around the house, but we were committed to a six-month lease. I aired out the house as much as I could for the three days I was there and left a few windows open. The landlord was sympathetic.

We arrived in Creemore a month later after the long drive from Dallas. I opened the front door of the house with some trepidation, which changed to resignation as we moved in our things. I knew Barbara wouldn't last long there. She made it through two nights after long days away from the house, then flew back to Dallas — wheezing, headachy, and miserable. It was annoying, inconvenient, expensive, and absolutely necessary that she get back to an environment that wouldn't stress her body any further.

An unsafe house can bring to mind desperate measures for those who can't tolerate the indoor environment. Before Barbara left, we discussed a number of possible 'fixes' to reduce the off-gassing. We finally focused on one obvious source of air pollution, the newly installed Ikea kitchen cabinets. We would treat them with AFM Hard Seal, a clear sealer that forms a membrane which prevents VOCs from outgassing. The landlord was skeptical, but gave us the go-ahead.

To its credit, Ikea has steadily reduced the amount of formaldehyde in its products over the past twenty years.[6] But the chemical is still used as a binder in its wood-based materials, such as particle board and plywood, in adhesives and lacquers, and as a finishing treatment on textiles like pillows and seat covers. Less is good, but for the chemically sensitive, even some is no good. My task was to prevent the off-gassing of the formaldehyde binders and glues by sealing every exposed surface of particle board—much of which was unseen under the counter top — as well as the hundreds of holes drilled through the laminate for adjustable shelves. All the interior laminate veneers also required sealing; we assumed the exteriors had off-gassed enough and didn't want to chance ruining the finish. More assumptions.

It was painstaking work. The laminate surfaces required sanding with 150-grit block then wiped down so the Hard Seal coat wouldn't sag — inside cupboards, all around drawers, under the sink, behind the dishwasher. Each hole for adjustable shelves was sealed using the only tool that made sense to me: a Q-Tip soaked in Hard Seal. In all, it was more than twenty hours of gymnastic work for a modestly sized kitchen.

It didn't help much. When Barbara returned from Dallas ten days later, the house was still off-gassing. We couldn't pin down what materials used in the renovation were the source. Motivated by her all-day headaches, draining sinuses, and almost continual coughing, the potential solutions became increasingly extreme. Seal all the kitchen cabinetry. Refinish the walls with a zero-VOC paint. Cover all the hardwood floors with a sealant to prevent off-gassing. Almost anything we thought of was wildly expensive, and seemed wildly indulgent for a short-term lease on someone else's property.

We had read in Dr. William Rea's book, *Optimum Environments for Optimum Health and Creativity*,[7] that high concentrations of formaldehyde occur in conditions of high temperature, high humidity and low air turnover. Our highly unscientific theory was that if we could create those conditions ourselves, we might be able to accelerate the off-gassing of the house. It was an unconventional solution but we were out of reasonable options. It was time for desperate measures.

We moved out to a bed and breakfast around the corner, returning to close up the house. Though it was 30C (86F) outside, we turned on the furnace and cranked the heat up to 38C or 100F — about as high as it would go. We would heat the house for 24 hours straight, then open all the windows, turn on the fans and ventilate for 12 hours.

We returned after the first 'bake-off' to a particularly noxious stew of off-gas from formaldehyde, paint, varnish, polyurethane and heating oil. But our theory seemed to be working. Ultimately, it took four heating-ventilating cycles — about one hundred hours of heating — and ongoing ventilation from open doors and windows to make the house livable for Barbara.

In previous chapters, we've talked about some of the strategies, systems, and materials we used to get the best possible indoor air quality in *+House*. In the context of looking for the unseen, it is most useful to detail the major approaches the design team used to avoid the most common problems associated with poor air quality in homes. It's worth noting that mold, humidity, and ventilation discussed below are closely related factors in any house and that it took a combination of design and systems to ensure we ended up with a comfortable, healthy house.[8]

Off-gassing of Materials. Off-gassing, or "out-gassing" as it is sometimes called, is the evaporation of synthetic chemicals — volatile organic compounds (VOCs) and semi-organic volatile compounds (SVOCs) — used in manufacturing. They are ubiquitous in our environment and can be found in products as varied as computer monitors, window blinds, automobile dashboards, mattresses, and cleaning products. In homes, four main categories of VOCs and SVOCs can pollute the indoor air quality: glued wood products, carpets, paints, and sealants, and furnishings treated with flame retardants or stain repellants. Depending on the age and health of a person's detoxification systems, exposure to these often-odorless substances can lead to asthma, allergies, fatigue, and memory loss. Prolonged exposure can lead to much worse. Formaldehyde, one of the most prevalent industrial chemicals (think of the smell of new cars, new carpets, and new cabinets), is a known human carcinogen at high exposures.[9]

The building team used a number of strategies to ensure *+House* had the best indoor air quality from the moment we moved in.

Walls / Wall Finishes. Standard construction typically specifies drywall and paint in new homes and renovations. But gypsum drywall is covered with recycled newspaper, which can off-gas residual VOCs from printing inks. Premixed joint compound may also contain formaldehyde and a variety of chemical dryers. Our eventual choice of Durisol block and American Clay, neither of which contain VOCs, eliminated this issue. All interior walls in the living space are clad in DensArmor Plus, a paperless drywall, and finished with smooth clay. There was no need for paint on the walls.

Millwork. Standard cabinetry construction and finishing is a prime source of VOCs. Cabinetry boxes or cases are usually made of particleboard, low-grade plywoods or melamine with a particleboard core; the majority of these substrates use formaldehyde-based glues. Even solid-wood doors or drawers are typically coated with solvent-based finishes. All of this contributes greatly to poor indoor air quality while the millwork is actively gassing off.

In Lesson 5, I described our strategy of heating the pre-finished millwork panels to accelerate off-gassing prior to fabrication and installation, as well as the necessity of sealing every hole needed for adjustable shelving and banding any exposed edges of the substrate. After installation, the supplier also used plugs to further seal any unused holes intended for adjustable shelf supports. The cumulative effect of this cautious approach was what we wanted — the house was immediately habitable for Barbara — but it was not perfect. Some of the large cabinets along the north wall were still obviously off-gassing when we opened the doors. The only solution was to keep the cabinet doors open, along with the windows and skylights, whenever we would be out of the house for a day. In other words, ventilate the off-gasses.

Wood Finishes and Sealants. Just three materials make up the primary components the living space of *+House*— concrete, wood and clay. The American Clay, as noted, does not off-gas. Wood was a different matter. In addition to the strategy for the millwork described in the last chapter, we needed one for the clear cedar to be installed on the ceiling, as Barbara had reacted to the sample. Since cedar is an aromatic wood, it was coated — to very nice effect — with AFM Safecoat Acrylaq satin sealant, which locks-in the wood's natural off-gassing. Similarly, the oak forming the interior side of the doors and windows was also finished with AFM Safecoat Hard Seal, a formula that prevents off-gassing from less-porous surfaces. The concrete was treated with Acri-Soy clear satin sealant to protect it from spills and stains.

Paint. Painters had very little work to do at *+House*. Just three doors and trim in the front hall called for a paint finish, as did the two-inch baseboard throughout the house. Those components were painted off-site and then installed. The cold-rolled steel mantle was also painted. In all cases, Superkül specified Safecoat zero-VOC paints.

Furnishings. While we worked with Marianne McKenna, our consulting architect, on the style and color palette for the furniture, it was up to us to make the selection as healthy as possible. That's a challenge with furniture, which can be manufactured with materials like flame retardants, formaldehyde-based glues, synthetic foams and plywood or particleboard. These materials can out-gas for years, and that presents a potentially serious risk for the chemically sensitive (and the long-term health of everyone else).

It was a lengthy search for the right combination of style and construction, with no North American manufacturers meeting the high bar we had set. (Admittedly, there was a degree of vanity in this process. We would soon have a cool contemporary home and wanted furnishings to match, though not at a price to our health.) We eventually chose pieces by Flexform and Molteni from Italy, and Ligne Roset from France,[10] and took a leap of faith that the higher European standards for clean manufacturing, water-based glues and minimal off-gassing would meet our needs. As a precaution, we ordered the furniture well in advance of installation so that it could be stored uncovered in local warehouses to air out. As we said in an email to the supplier, "Received the furniture last Thursday, and it looks (and smells) great."

Because the polished concrete floors are a major design feature of +*House*, we had no intention of covering them with broadloom (and all the chemical soup that typically entails). We do use area rugs — mostly synthetic materials with little out-gas — in the living room and guest and master bedrooms to help define those areas and offer some warmth underfoot when the floor is cooler.

Wait, There's More!

Minimizing off-gassing materials is not the only factor needed for healthy indoor air quality. Dealing proactively with potential issues from mold, humidity, ventilation, and products of combustion are also very important considerations in achieving an optimal living environment.

Mold Growth. Mold, left untreated, can bring with it a whole host of nasty health risks, including symptoms like eye, nose and throat irritation, wheezing and shortness of breath, and worsening of asthma.[11] It was clear to everyone on the design team that as many factors as possible that could contribute to dampness and mold would have to be mitigated. There would be no basement—a big loss of potential space but a bigger risk for high humidity and mold. And rerouting the flow of water from the hill behind the house would be essential. "A big concern for us," André said, "was ensuring we could divert the water. We were able to manage that quite easily with high and low layers of weeping tile and lots of granular fill. We wanted to make sure there was no pressure on the house from the water coming off the hill."

With the north, east and west sides of the house well-drained, and the south side a window wall from which rain drains easily to the pond, we have had no issues with unintended water or mold. Inside the house, we've taken normal precautions to ensure all water lines are well connected. The mechanical room, which houses the water furnace, hot water tanks, washing machine and water conditioning equipment, is one area of vulnerability. A high-water alarm in the low point of the space connected to our home monitoring system has on at least one occasion proven to be a very useful and inexpensive addition.

Ventilation Issues. Following on the oil crises of the 1970s came stricter building standards for homes that were intended to improve energy efficiency. The natural ventilation that came from less rigorous construction methods and materials — literally, "leaky houses" — was effectively eliminated to reduce energy usage, but that strategy typically led to airtight and poorly ventilated spaces. While less costly to run, these homes left their occupants vulnerable to the health effects of biological and chemical pollutants such as mold, pollens, dust mites, products of combustion (furnace, gas stove, cigarettes), and off-gassing of volatile organic compounds from building materials, cleaning products, and furniture. Few building codes mandate sufficient turnover of indoor air to eliminate these pollutants from our living spaces.

+*House* was certainly designed to be airtight and energy efficient. Ensuring it would also be healthy required a ventilation strategy that was both passive and intentional. Passive air flow is a key feature of the design. Ventilation from six very large screen doors — nine feet high by seven feet wide — across the south side is augmented by five smaller operable windows, as well as by operating windows on the east and west sides of the house. Windows along the north wall also open to allow air flow from the cooler forested area behind the house. Warmer air can be exhausted through three operating skylights — two in the main living space and one over the master bathroom. Ceiling fans help keep the air moving on still days.

Because it is used year-round, the house is ducted for supplemental heat and air-conditioning. "We wanted to use the ventilation system primarily for cooling," André told me, "so we have the ducts up high so you get even distribution of cool air as it drops. The slab is heated by geothermal energy, the main source of heating, but you can also use the supplemental heat of the furnace through the ducts. Our main goal was that the cross-ventilation would be sufficient to cool on most days, and on the hot, humid, still days you can turn on the air-conditioning." We upgraded to heat-mirror, triple glazing throughout the house to help reduce the need for air-conditioning on all but the most hot, humid days.

With the windows and doors open, air exchange is not an issue. But there are many days during the year when the house is closed up, which required an intention to keep the living space well-ventilated and free of pollutants. Superkül's solution was to build a ventilation system that combined a heat recovery ventilator (HRV) with a whole house air cleaner.

HRVs are a great appliance for modern, airtight homes because they pull fresh outside air into the home at the same time they exhaust stale air. And as the two air flows pass in separate chambers, the unit transfers heating or cooling from the outgoing air to the fresh air, which in turn reduces energy costs. In *+House*, conditioned fresh air then passes through a Lifebreath TFP air cleaner. The Lifebreath unit runs continuously, operating on a principle known as "turbulent flow precipitation" that uses the airflow to move particles into a cleanable collection space. This, combined with a downstream HEPA (high-efficiency particulate air) filter, cleans the air of effectively 99.9 percent of airborne particles before sending it back into the ventilation system. A "hospital-grade" system, as Superkül described it.

High / Low Humidity. Regulating the amount of humidity in our living space is an important factor of our overall comfort and health.[12] We add to ambient levels by our myriad human activities — breathing, cooking, showering, laundry. We deplete it by heating and cooling, especially in today's airtight homes. Too much humidity can lead to issues such as condensation on windows, moldy bathrooms, and a musty smell. Too little can result in static electricity, chapped skin, and breathing problems.

Conventionally built homes, with their paint-over-drywall-over-vapor-barrier construction, typically require supplementary humidification in winter to maintain optimum relative humidity. And, to be honest, that type of interior construction was what had been initially specified for *+House*, albeit with healthier materials. It was our visit with Robert Stellar, the building biologist, who introduced us to the remarkable properties of the two building products detailed in the last chapter — Durisol block and American Clay.

Our decision to use Durisol in the perimeter walls was based primarily on its 'breathability.' A breathable wall system is "diffusion open and hygroscopic," according to the manufacturer. That means it allows water vapor to be absorbed during periods of high humidity and slowly released when the humidity is lower — what's called humidity buffering. By Durisol's measurements,[13] coating its wall system with an earthen plaster like clay or lime provides indoor vapor control nearly 15 times greater than painted gypsum drywall.

American Clay is a key part of this vapor control. We've all seen water droplets form on painted walls after a hot shower on a cold day. This happens to varying degree throughout a house when there is excess humidity — think condensation on windows. Clay plaster, by contrast, absorbs water before it can form into droplets, significantly reducing the potential for mold and mildew growth. When the humidity drops throughout the house, the American Clay releases moisture into the living space to help keep the humidity constant. Because the walls act as the "lungs" of the house, breathing in and breathing out, we've never needed a humidifier to keep +*House* comfortable during winter heating.

Superkül also specified a mechanical means of controlling excess moisture. While the HRV is always on, its exhaust power can be boosted in the bathrooms to eliminate vapor and odors; standalone exhaust fans augment the air extraction. The control system of the HRV also allows us to control the relative humidity in the house. We set it to 45 percent in winter and have had no issues with condensation on cold surfaces. An important lesson we learned about this control feature of HRVs is that it should be set to zero during the months when the air conditioning is on. If it's not, you will be pulling in humid outside air at the same time the air-conditioning unit is trying to dehumidify the house — not energy efficient!

Products of Combustion. There are two primary sources of particles and gases that can pollute the indoor environment in a home — cooking and heating. Smoking is a third, but that kind of lifestyle choice begs the question of why bother building a healthy house when you're intent on crippling a healthy body.

As we discovered years earlier when Barbara was at her most chemically sensitive, gas stoves — responsive as they are to cook on — throw off nitrogen dioxide, carbon monoxide, and formaldehyde as the natural gas burns.[14] Even with a powerful exhaust fan, there was sufficient residual pollution that she became unable to tolerate using the cooktop, and we reluctantly switched to an electric range. The choice for +*House*, then, was simple: an electric stovetop and oven. Not that we had the option of natural gas lines running by the property.

The undesirability of gas or propane dictated the choice of heating for the house. The primary source of heating is in-floor hydronic radiant heat. The heat is derived from the in–pond geothermal loops and extracted by the water furnace, then pumped through a closed system of tubing set in the concrete slab. Supplemental heat and air-conditioning are electric — no products of combustion there and no concerns about carbon monoxide buildup that can result from poorly vented gas- or oil-burning furnaces.

We debated at some length about the wisdom of installing a fireplace. Wood smoke, according to the EPA, contains toxic harmful air pollutants that include particulates, benzene, formaldehyde, acrolein, and polycyclic aromatic hydrocarbons (PAHs).[15] Backdrafts can cause smoke from a fire to push out into the room, making life miserable for days for the chemically sensitive or those with breathing issues. But the shoulder seasons and long winters of Ontario almost demanded the warmth of a hearth if we could find a model that reduced the risk of backdrafts. We eventually settled on a Belgian-made Stüv fireplace. It was more expensive to buy and install than many we looked at, but has many excellent features for our needs — its own outside air supply, precise control of air volume and burn rate, self-cleaning front glass, and abundant heating capability. We've never been smoked out of the house. That said, individuals with concerns about products of combustion in their living environment can always install a computer monitor with the sound and image of a crackling fire and substitute LED candles for the real thing. Thanks to Mark Cree Jackson for the suggestions.

The core ideas of building healthy could be summarized as a combination of what you put in and what you keep out. In our experience, it was easier and more interesting to identify the elements that went into the physical house — the design, building materials, finishes — than it was to discover the unseen things that should be kept out — mold, excess humidity, EMF, off-gasses. But it's the acknowledgement that both efforts are necessary for success that will ultimately determine how healthy the house will be for its occupants.

In the case of +*House*, the open spaces, expansive views, and the feeling of 'softness' that the clay walls impart are integral to the experience of living there. But so is the unseen 'softness' that comes the movement of air, the minimal EMF, and the freedom from chemical burden. Our bodies are given a space to relax and re-generate, freed from the overloads they must navigate in more conventional environments.

That's our measure of success.

Notes

1   Electricity is deemed "dirty" when the original 60 Hz power is contaminated by high-frequency signals emanating from an overloaded electrical distribution system and from computers, routers, and other appliances. Microsurges related to dirty electricity can be reduced by Stetzerizer filters -- **http://www.stetzerelectric.com** – which we use in our Dallas house. The research, however, is contentious. A contrary view is briefly summarized at **http://www.radiationsafety.ca/the-truth-about-dirty-electricity**

2   In 2011, the International Agency for Research on Cancer, an agency of the World Health Organization, issued summary of its findings titled, "IARC classifies radiofrequency electromagnetic fields as possibly carcinogenic to humans." The study cited increased risk of gliomas, a malignant type of brain cancer, associated with long-term wireless phone use. You can find an overview of the research and links to more information at **http://www.iarc.fr/en/media-centre/pr/2011/pdfs/pr208_E.pdf**. IARC's findings, needless to say, are at odds with studies funded by the mobile communications industry.

3   From the Health Canada website: **http://www.hc-sc.gc.ca/hl-vs/iyh-vsv/prod/meters-compteurs-eng.php**. To their credit, Health Canada also cited the IARC paper in the footnote above.

4   Available on the U.S. Federal Communications Commission website at: **http://apps.fcc.gov/ecfs/document/view%3Bjsession-id%3DNDTPRSrKjyXK9QsNy4w9vdqyDnJBZz-wSLn065qWb2M12LXjq122s!956499833!NONE%-3Fid%3D7022118538**.

5   See **http://smartmeterguard.com**.

6   **http://www.naturalstep.org/en/usa/ikea**

7   Rea, Dr. William, *Optimum Environments for Optimum Health and Creativity: Designing and Building a Healthy Home or Office*. Self-published, Environmental Health Center, Dallas, Texas.

8   The EPA offers excellent construction specifications, called "Indoor AirPLUS", that are designed to achieve optimal indoor air quality. See   **http://www.epa.gov/indoorairplus/advantages-and-fea-tures-indoor-airplus-homes#features**.

9   **http://www.atsdr.cdc.gov/substances/toxsubstance.asp?tox-id=39**

10   These manufacturers are noted for their high quality of design and construction and their products are priced accordingly. For a comprehensive discussion of options for healthy furnishings, see *Prescriptions for a Healthy House*, 3rd edition, pp.189-201.

11   Health   Canada   **http://healthycanadians.gc.ca/healthy-living-vie-saine/environment-environnement/air/contaminants/mould-moisissures-eng.php**. See also the Environmental Protection Agency's guide to mold in the home at **http://www.epa.gov/mold/brief-guide-mold-moisture-and-your-home**.

12   A good general discussion of humidity and its measurement can be found at **http://publications.gc.ca/collections/collection_2011/schl-cmhc/nh18-24/NH18-24-1-2009-eng.pdf**.

13   **http://durisolbuild.com/Webdocs/DurisolIAQ.pdf**

14   For an interesting review of some of the science, see "Cooking Up Indoor Air Pollution: Emissions from Natural Gas Stoves." From *Environmental Health Perspectives* published by the National Institute of Environmental Health Sciences. **http://ehp.niehs.nih.gov/122-a27/**

15   **https://www.epa.gov/burnwise/wood-smoke-and-your-health**

Keeping It
(and Yourself) Healthy

In the previous chapters, I have described at length the many decisions we made, and the many reasons motivating them, to ensure that we didn't introduce potentially harmful chemicals and frequencies into *+House* while it was being built and furnished. But then we moved in and took on the familiar rhythms and habits of everyday living. What did we have to do to ensure we kept the indoor environment and air quality as healthy as possible?

Thanks largely to effective marketing, we modern consumers tend to be brand conscious and brand loyal. And in the absence of some compelling alternative in our busy lives, we stick with what works, we stick with what's familiar, and we stick with what's well-priced, especially for everyday commodities. But this stick-with-it mindset has the potential to be damaging to our health and particularly debilitating for the chemically sensitive person.

Recall that in Lesson 1 I referred to the approximately 80,000 chemicals currently in use, 99 percent of which have never been tested for their effects on human health. Compared to the relatively simple, often natural ingredients used just a couple of generations ago, the products we buy today for household cleaning and personal care are largely complex synthetic formulas devised by the specialty chemical industry. As the authors of *Slow Death by Rubber Duck* put it, "… it's been estimated that by the time the average woman grabs her morning coffee, she has applied 126 different chemicals in 12 different products to her face, body and hair."[1] With the growing popularity (and advertising) of men's care products, men can't be far behind. And that's before either starts cleaning the house.[2]

Mainstream household cleaning products can be a poorly disclosed amalgam of potentially toxic ingredients that none of us, let alone those who may be dealing with chemical overload already, should breath in or come in contact with. Volatile organic compounds, formaldehyde, dyes, fragrances, phthalates, antibacterials, stain repellents — to name only a handful of thousands of possible offenders — have been linked to a host of ailments that include some forms of cancer, reproductive issues, respiratory illnesses and developmental disorders.

If this sounds alarmist, visit the Environmental Working Group's *Guide to Healthy Cleaning*, an online database that enables you to search their analysis and ratings of more than 2,000 cleaning products.[3] Rankings range from "A, Lowest Concern: Few / no known or suspected hazards to health or the environment. Good ingredient disclosure" to "F, Highest Concern: Potentially significant hazards to health or the environment or poor ingredient disclosure." According to the EWG, "the ratings indicate the relative level of concern posed by exposure to the ingredients in this product — not the product itself — compared with other product formulations. Given that context, consider EWG's ratings and summary commentary on four well-known household products:

- **Bounce™ Dryer Sheets**. Rating: D. "May contain ingredients with potential for respiratory effects; nervous system effects; skin irritation / allergies / damage."

- **Febreze™ Fabric Refresher**. Rating: F. "May contain ingredients with potential for developmental / endocrine / reproductive effects; acute aquatic toxicity; respiratory effects."

- **Palmolive™ Ultra Dish Liquid, Original**. Rating: F. "May contain ingredients with potential for cancer; respiratory effects; damage to vision." for developmental / endocrine / reproductive effects; respiratory effects; biodegradation."

- **Windex™ Foaming Glass Cleaner**. Rating: F. "May contain ingredients with potential for developmental / endocrine / reproductive effects; acute aquatic toxicity; respiratory effects."

While EWG's *Guide* cannot specify how much exposure to these ingredients it might take to produce these health effects in specific individuals, it should make any consumer think seriously about the wisdom of using products like these at all, particularly if that consumer is experiencing health issues that may be — or already are — related to toxic overload. With a little research, you will discover there are many good alternatives. One particularly useful feature of the EWG site is the ability to easily find healthier, more environmentally friendly substitutes for mainstream products. A single click on the Windex™ page noted above, for example, turned up nine A-rated alternatives.

Making the Necessary Choices

Our own path to using healthier cleaning options began well before *+House* was completed. We described in chapter one how Barbara came to know, in 2002, that her body's internal detoxification system was not fully functioning. An important part of the strategy to help her reduce that bodily load was to eliminate as many new potential toxins as we could in our living environment. Cleaning products and fragrances were at the top of the list.

When Barbara began treatment at the Environmental Health Center in Dallas (EHCD) in 2006, the need to stay clear of chemical exposures was critical. Even the fragrances she encountered during a walk around the neighborhood on laundry day could upset her body chemistry and compromise both the testing and treatment protocols. It was at the EHCD that Barbara met Carolyn Gorman, an environmental consultant and the author of *Less-Toxic Alternatives*, a book that dramatically deepened our understanding of what it meant, and what it took, to live a truly healthier lifestyle. Now in its tenth edition,[4] *Less-Toxic Alternatives* remains our touchstone when we need practical guidance about virtually any household and personal care issue. We highly recommend it.

Over the years since our awareness of environmental chemicals had begun to grow, we had evolved a home and personal 'maintenance' regime that worked for us. And though there are some differences between products available in Canada versus the United States, it was relatively easy to adopt it at our new home. The key words here are "worked for us." It's a process of trial and error that depends on your sensitivities. Our preference for natural products, some with essential oil fragrances, may not work for everyone. There are many alternatives now available, increasingly at mainstream grocery chains. If you have one in your area, "natural" grocery stores like Whole Foods typically have a good selection of natural cleaning and paper products.

With the caveat to find the products that work best for you, here's what we use to ensure we keep +*House* as healthy as possible. One note: overall, these products rate quite well on the EWG database mentioned above. An exception was the 4X laundry detergent, which rated a "D." The unconcentrated, powdered version of the same product ranked an "A" and is a healthier, though less convenient, choice.

Kitchen

- Seventh Generation™ Natural Dish Liquid, Free & Clear (scent)

- Seventh Generation™ Natural Glass & Surface Cleaner, Free & Clear

- Seventh Generation™ Natural Dishwasher Detergent, Free & Clear

- Seventh Generation™ Rinse Aid

Bathrooms

- Seventh Generation™ Natural All-purpose Cleaner, Free & Clear

- Seventh Generation™ Natural Tub & Tile Cleaner, Emerald Cypress & Fir

- Seventh Generation™ Natural Toilet Bowl Cleaner, Emerald Cypress & Fir

Laundry

- Seventh Generation™ 4X Natural Laundry Detergent, Free & Clear

- Seventh Generation™ Chlorine-Free Bleach, Free & Clear

- Ecover™ Natural Stain Remover

- Ecover™ Delicate Wash

Windows

- Seventh Generation™ Natural Dish Liquid

Pesticides. In Dallas, many homeowners use pesticides inside and out to keep critters like spiders, fire ants, earwigs, scorpions and roaches at bay. While there are some formulations that use naturally derived ingredients, the most widely used pesticides contain organophosphates and organochlorides that can affect numerous body systems, especially the brain. These are dangerous chemicals that have no place in a healthy home or garden, and we do not use them. We have come to a peaceful co-existence with the insects and animals that also call our property home and, despite no pesticide use, we have had no issues in or around +*House* that were other than minimally inconvenient. When necessary, we apply Orange Guard™ Home Pest Control, a citrus-based spray pesticide. But that use has admittedly been limited to moderate northern climates that do not have the same intensity of bugs or heat that the South experiences.

The Ultimate Cleaning Product

I've made no mention so far about the water system we installed in the house. Yet clean water, free of chemical and organic contaminants, is absolutely essential, not just for a clean house but also for the health of our bodies.

Being in the country, the water source for +*House* is a drilled well. Our installer found the best combination of water quality and flow rates was from 165 feet, and that's where he capped the well. After entering the house, the untreated water flows through dual sediment filters and then into an ultraviolet filter to eliminate bacteria. Titration tests showed that the water coming from the well was quite hard, so we elected to install a salt-based softener (though we set the salt usage to its minimum level). There was also a sulphurous taste and odor to the well water, which the supplier attributed to "organic iron." To remediate that issue, we opted for a standalone iron filter — a chemical-free system in which fresh air provides the oxidation needed to remove the contaminants.

Because the original house had a dug well and some filtration equipment of questionable effectiveness, during our one summer there we installed a reverse osmosis system in the kitchen to ensure we had good drinking water. We put the system in storage during construction, then reinstalled it in the kitchen, with an additional line to the ice-cube maker in the freezer.

Just before our site supervisor, Jeff Pepper, was going to start up the finished water system, we received an email from him on an aspect of new construction we had never considered:

> [The supplier] is onsite finishing off the water treatment system. I had to stop him from super-chlorinating the system because I wanted to discuss this part of the process with you. Our technician mentioned that he fills up the sediment filter with chlorine and then runs that through all the plumbing. This will have to be done just before occupancy but I was hoping there was another more eco-friendly liquid that

we could use or if it was a concern to Barbara at all. Please let me know your feelings on this.

Barbara's feelings were strong and immediate. Chlorine is a potent chemical; we didn't even use chlorine bleach for laundry. While flushing water systems with chlorine may be the industry standard, the supplier had successfully used hydrogen peroxide for the task, which is what they used to prepare our system.

Clean by Design (and Intent)

During the initial design presentations, we had been impressed with how concerned Superkül was about trying to ensure that we could keep the house free of dust, mold, and other allergens. As the design, especially of the millwork, came into its final form, we could see that maintaining +*House* would be relatively simple. There was to be minimal open shelving, and where it was open it was mostly at a level within easy reach. All cupboards and cabinets would not only be closed but also integrated into walls to eliminate dust-gathering surfaces. Our commitment was to limit the amount of "stuff" around the house without making it feel like an upscale hotel room — a few books, some family photos, one or two treasures. All easily cleaned, and cleaned around.

As I've described, one of the innovative design features of +*House* is its strategy for passive ventilation.

Windows along the north wall bring in cooler air from the forest to the north; the skylights exhaust warmer air. Depending on the temperature, we can use smaller, screened windows on the south side or open the huge screened doors to feel like we're in an enclosed porch. As great as this sounds for air flow, it's also great for dust and pollen flow. So during those seasons when the HRV and Lifebreath air filter can't quite keep up to the standards Barbara needs for her comfort, additional cleaning, or closing up the house, is sometimes necessary.

I have tried to make the point throughout this book that the design, materials, and systems that go into healthy building are quite personal. They should be derived to meet the specific needs of the occupants. Someone with electromagnetic hypersensitivity may build a very different house, in a different location, than someone whose main issue is multiple chemical sensitivity or a compromised immune system. The same specificity should extend to keeping the living environment clean and healthy.

With that in mind, what follows is *our* cleaning regimen. It is not to say how or when *you* should clean your home to keep it healthy for your needs. Rather, it is a schedule that enables us to feel as well as possible in our home given our distinct needs.

Weekly
- Dust all accessible surfaces with damp, lint-free cloth.

- HEPA vacuum floors, area rugs, furniture.

- Clean bathrooms and kitchen, damp-mop floors.

Monthly
- Dust cabinet door tops, ventilation grates, etc.

- Dust lamp shades and lights.

- Damp-mop all concrete floors.

Twice a year
- Clean windows inside and out.

- Clean top windowsills, uplights.

- Dust closet and cabinet interiors.

If all of this seems relatively simple, it is, and intentionally so. There are many things other than cleaning that we enjoy doing in and around +*House*. But this is such an important part of the overall healthiness of the house that just missing a weekly clean can lead to days of headaches and congestion for Barbara. We have a system and try our best to stick to it for the simple satisfaction of feeling well in a living environment built for that very purpose.

Notes

1   Smith, Rick and Lourie, Bruce, *Slow Death by Rubber Duck: The Secret Danger of Everyday Things*. Counterpoint Press, Berkeley, CA. Kindle Edition. p.3.

2   If you are concerned about the safety of personal care products and cosmetics you're using, I suggest you consult a new Environmental Working Group service called Skin Deep®. According to the website, to earn the EWG VERIFIEDTM logo, products must avoid ingredients of concern, provide full transparency and use good manufacturing process. You will find the site at **http://www.ewg.org/skindeep/search.php?ewg_verified=introduction**.

3   **http://www.ewg.org/guides/cleaners**. With regard to its ratings, EWG states: "EWG provides information on cleaning product ingredients from the published scientific literature, to supplement incomplete data available from companies and the government. The ratings indicate the relative level of concern posed by exposure to the ingredients in this product — not the product itself — compared to other product formulations. The ratings reflect potential health hazards but do not account for the level of exposure or individual susceptibility, factors which determine actual health risks, if any."

4   Gorman, Carolyn, *Less-Toxic Alternatives*. Tenth Edition, Optimum Publishing, 2010. Available from Amazon or the American Environmental Health Foundation (www.AEHF.com), Dallas, TX.

Lesson 8:

Healthy Is Holistic

It was never our specific intention to build a so-called "green" house. Our focus had always been on building as healthy a home as possible. If less green had meant healthier, we would have opted for healthy. And on more than one occasion, especially when it came to using materials with recycled content, that was a choice we were required to make. But the further we got along in the project, the more we — along with Superkül and Jeff Pepper — realized that green and healthy follow much the same path toward common goals like conserving energy, improving air quality, and minimizing environmental impact.

We had done our best from the start to protect the context in which the house would sit. With the property situated in the middle of a World Biosphere Preserve, we felt we should go beyond what was mandated if we could match our resources to our intention. We transplanted five, twenty-five-foot Nootka cypress trees prior to the beginning of construction, and other specimens were re-moved to a nursery for eventual replanting. The few trees we did need to take down for safety purposes during construction were mostly reforested red pines nearing the end of their natural lives. The useful parts from the old house had been salvaged by the local Habitat for Humanity crew, and the demolition contractor ensured that what could be recycled was. We even relocated the bat house from the side of the original house to the hill above the site in the hope that they would continue to keep the area around the pond free from insects. (Sadly, the bats moved elsewhere.)

We had made other "green" decisions without any real awareness that the cumulative impact might be important. Early on, we elected to install a high-tech EcoFlo septic system because it enabled us to keep the old system in place — less material to landfills — leave dozens of trees and bushes untouched, and avoid a signif-icant amount of new, non-native fill required to rebuild a standard-size field. The in-pond geothermal system also lessens the environmental impact of the house. Because it uses the differential in temperature between the water at the bottom of the pond and the outside air to augment heating and cooling cycles, it reduces energy usage. The green roof adds an insulating layer to the house that also lowers energy consumption while it helps control storm-water runoff.

It was when the realization dawned that we had made a lot of good decisions about the health of our immediate environment that we began the discussion of the possibility of LEED certification for +*House*.

Barbara and I had certainly heard of the LEED designation but we weren't sure it was relevant to what we were trying to accomplish in building a *healthy* house. LEED is an acronym for Leadership in Energy and Environmental Design, "an internationally accepted benchmark for the design, construction and operation of high-performance green buildings," according to the Canada Green Building Council.[1] LEED Canada for Homes, like its counterpart in the United States, uses third-party raters to certify green homes using criteria in eight very detailed categories; all projects must meet nineteen mandatory measures. Homes are given either a Certified, Silver, Gold or Platinum rating — Platinum being the "greenest" dwelling — based on points awarded in five key areas of human and environmental well-being: sustainable site development, water efficiency, energy efficiency, materials selection, and indoor environmental quality.

As the house moved towards completion by mid-2011, any LEED statement we wanted to make about water use, energy efficiency, materials selection, and indoor environmental quality had already been made. But with the growing awareness that LEED certification at some level was likely, we wondered what more we could reasonably do that was in keeping with our intention to be healthy. "Sustainable site development" was the one measure we could still influence, so we turned our attention outwards, to the areas around the house. We obviously had to create a new landscape following construction. How could we do it better?

Like the design of +*House*, and for some of the same reasons, the landscaping was an evolution. We had hired a well-regarded local landscape architect and contractor and briefed them on our limited budget and preference for a natural, easy-to-maintain look. The plan we eventually received was well-integrated and arguably appropriate to the house, with about 150 feet of gabion wall to retain the back hill and an equal length of reinforced concrete wall set at various right angles across the front of the deck to hold back that even-steeper slope. There were abundant plantings behind the house and right down to the pond, where the designers envisioned a new deck and dock.

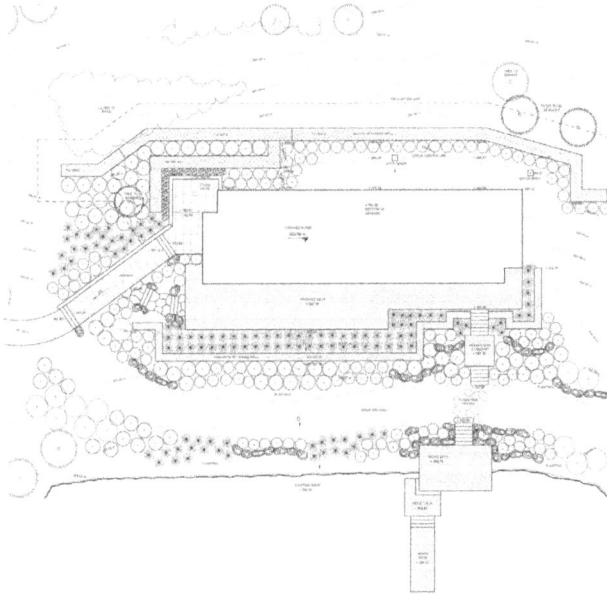

Not exactly what we had in mind for the landscaping.

The plan, however, bore a similarity to the first version of designs we saw for the house — exciting to contemplate and expensive to realize. Even by postponing the pond deck and (somehow) the plantings, the cost to construct doubled the budget for all of the landscape work. And it would introduce a huge amount of new rock and concrete to the site where there had been little before and necessitate hauling in large amounts of fill. As we said in an email to Jeff after reviewing the plans, "While we like the overall concept... it seems 'over-designed' to us...

We would like a simple solution, especially for the back, that is in keeping with the rural context and the design of the house, and which will drain well enough to keep the hill intact and the house dry." The landscape designers apparently did not agree with our preferences or weren't willing to put a professional stamp on a more-natural and less-expensive solution. We parted ways.

It was mid-March — with a midsummer finish promised — and we were back at square one. We were in Dallas, and, as Jeff Pepper later recalled, "Landscaping was something I really didn't understand. It was a horrible issue for me to try to deal with." But as he had done throughout the project whenever he faced a challenge with materials, Jeff got on the computer and trolled the Internet, this time to find a better option for securing the back hill, which had by now become our first priority. We were all concerned that a few heavy spring rains might cause the soil to cascade down the slope and into the back of the house.

Jeff eventually discovered a product he called Envirolok bags, or what the manufacturer calls "Envirolok Ecological Engineered Solutions." Their marketing materials stated that "Envirolok has demonstrated appeal where immediate structural stability and integrity is required and a vegetated outcome is desired."[2] These were the right words, as far as we were concerned.

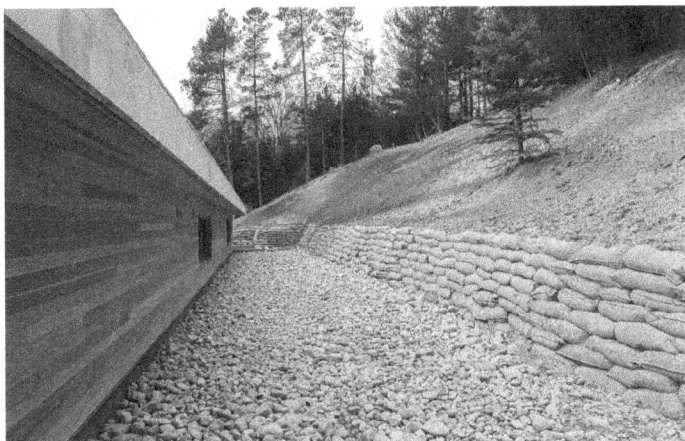

The graded slope with the Envirolok bags and river rock in place. The area had just been hydroseeded with grasses and wildflowers.

Barbara in particular had envisioned a broad expanse of wildflowers blanketing the hill, not the rock and wire mesh wall that had been proposed. The recycled-fiber bags seemed like the more-natural, cost-effective and greener solution we wanted.

Jeff produced a rudimentary but inspired sketch based on his growing instinct for landscape design. (I am keeping my promise not to reproduce it.) He proposed a wall of Envirolok bags, running parallel to the house. More bags would protect the exposed roots of trees near the top of the slope. The entire area, including the Envirolok wall, would be hydroseeded with fast-growing plants to secure the surface soil. Superkül weighed in with a few additional suggestions. Although it would not qualify for a landscape architect's stamp, we finally had a plan we could live with, at least for that part of the project. And it was a whole lot "greener" than the more professional options.

"Thank God for Martin Zeng and his boys" was a comment we heard from Jeff several times as the landscaping progressed. We echoed the sentiment too on numerous occasions. Jeff had hired Zeng Landscaping from nearby Creemore to make the back hill more "manageable," a euphemism for not so precipitously steep. Beginning at the top of the slope, Martin reshaped an old trail so that rainwater and snow melt from the forest would drain west to the road rather than down the hill to the house. Then began, we were told, a gravity-defying dance of the machines that reduced the pitch of the slope and moved soil to where it was needed. Using materials from the site to help stabilize the hill was not only environmentally friendly, it also eliminated the costly and by now logistically impossible alternative of bringing in truckloads of new fill.

With the basic contours established, Jeff and the Zeng team began filling the Envirolok bags with a mix of local soil and compost. The crew painstakingly built a four-foot high retaining wall that spanned more than 130 feet from the west side of the house until it tapered off around the east side. A French drain was set in the ten feet between the house and wall as a first defense against heavy runoff—two other lines were already installed at different depths along the back wall—and that entire area lined with river rock. With the Envirolok bags creating a solid "toe" for the slope, Zeng finalized the grade with fill from the sides of the hill. In early May, the entire area was hydroseeded with native wildflowers and grasses to stabilize the surface soil.

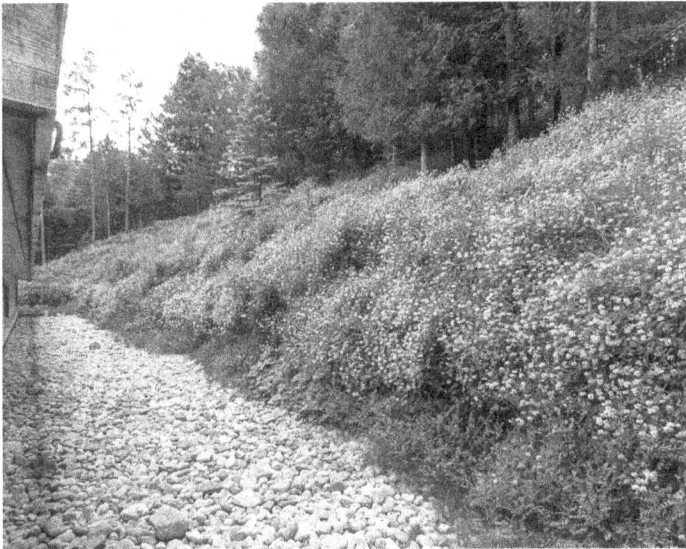

The back hill after grow-in.

During the weeks that followed, Zeng's Bobcat and mini-excavator roamed over the rest of the site, setting the slope of the front hill, establishing the pathway across the edge of the pond and leveling the small area that would become our "front lawn." We now had grades, but only a general idea of what should be planted. We held onto a guiding principle that whatever we did should be both sustainable and affordable. In our simplistic view of landscape design, we thought we could achieve "sustainable" if the plantings were local and perennial and wouldn't require huge commitments of time, water, and fertilizer to maintain. It's also true that our vision of sustainability had expanded beyond plants to include other materials used in creating the walkways, paths, and the driveway. "Affordable" certainly referred to the initial cost, but not necessarily the lowest cost. Given the substantial investment we had already made, we wanted uncomplicated, attractive landscaping that would enhance the house and its immediate context. We had no intention of reprising the beautiful, but very labor-intensive country gardens created by the previous owners.

Our sole design idea, a borrowed one at that, involved planting a geometric pattern of grasses across the front hill. We knew we also had a half-dozen small trees to bring back from the nursery, but where to replant them? What about some privacy while we were sitting on the deck? How would we stabilize the front hill? We needed help with design and execution. Zeng demurred on the planning work, not considering himself a designer, so we began to ask friends in the area to recommend someone who could help us create the outdoor palette we vaguely had in mind.

The consensus choice was a master gardener named Sherry Wilson, who lived in Creemore. I had known Sherry and her husband, David, years before, but had lost touch with them during my many moves. It was a very welcome reunion for us because Sherry not only understands the subtleties of country gardening, she also has boundless energy and a real vision for what is possible. Most importantly, she listened to what we wanted to accomplish in the name of simplicity and sustainability. It was another instance of having a 'serendipitous accomplice' join our team.

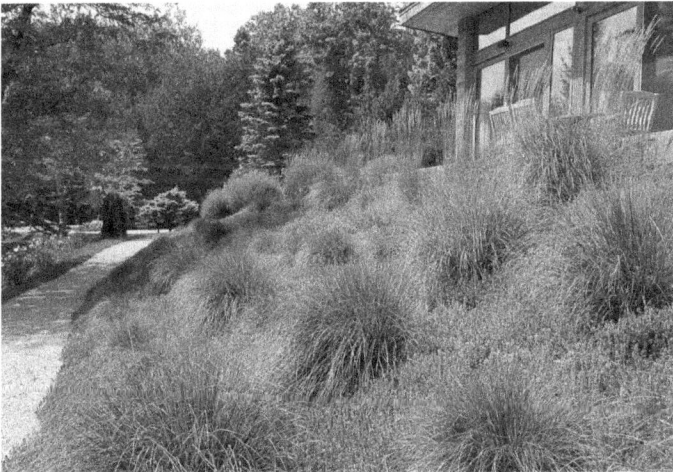

Thyme and ornamental grasses stabilize the front hill.

A few days after our initial meeting at the house, Sherry returned with a hand-sketched plan. We loved it. We would have our geometric pattern of ornamental grasses on the front hill, but there would also be a line of taller "Karl Foerster" grasses along the front of the deck to provide a visual barrier to the slope. Fast-growing Arctic willow bushes would be planted in the sight-line from the road to the deck. Then the entire graded area fronting the deck would be hydroseeded with organic compost and thyme seed — the same thyme that might be used in preparing a winter stew or savory pasta. It would grow quickly to stabilize the slope, self-seed each year, and require minimal maintenance. While the thyme and grasses were taking root, a recycled mesh 'sock' filled with organic compost would line the edge of the hill to prevent runoff of soil into the gravel walkway. The balance of the property not yet seeded would also receive a layer of organic compost and be hydroseeded with Eco-Lawn seed, a mixture of perennial rye grass and fescues that promised low-maintenance, low-water lawn areas.

The trees that had wintered in a local nursery were delivered — two smallish magnolias and four ornamental evergreens. Sherry had a general idea of where each tree should be located in the overall design but wanted to be sure each was positioned so that it would prosper. Not relying entirely on her own instinct, she 'dowsed' the exact placement of each tree. Now, if you've never seen dowsing performed, it can appear quite odd. Dowsing is a kind of divination tool that has been used for centuries to locate underground water or turn up lost items (or lost ways) or even answer arcane spiritual questions. The dowser holds a y-shaped branch or L-shaped metal rods or a small crystal on a short chain and asks questions — aloud or silently — to whatever may be their source of inspiration: the vast unknowables like intuition, the unconscious, the Universe, Spirit, God. Answers take a variety of forms depending on how the rods or pendulum move. It's all very individual and not what you would call scientific.

I had seen dowsing rods used on at least a couple of occasions to locate underground watercourses prior to well-drilling, and they worked. Whether they worked better than chance is impossible for the uninitiated to say. But as Sherry asked her questions and decoded the answers indicated by her pendulum, the placement of the trees gradually came into focus. It seemed like an ideal arrangement of elements to us, at least visually, and all but one of them gradually resumed their growth.

Our final landscaping decision was what to do about the hardscape on various parts of the property. We had decided on Eramosa limestone slabs for the front entrance area and steps down to the driveway grade; the same stone would be used for the steps down from the deck and to the dock. Martin Zeng assured us that a very good supplier was located about an hour west of us, near Wiarton, Ontario, and that their version of Eramosa, while not the most popular, had more visual character and better durability than the option that had to be transported all the way from Ohio.

The original house had had an expansive interlocking brick driveway connected to a path that meandered across the edge of the pond. The path was long gone, having been taken up with the demolition of the house. But after many months of traffic from heavy construction equipment, the driveway and parking area were a mess of wide ruts and broken bricks. The cost to remediate the problems was essentially the price of a new driveway, which was far too much to contemplate at that point.

The answer the team arrived at brought the ideas of "sustainable" and "affordable" together definitively. We would strip the brick and send it to a recycling facility. The driveway would be leveled, given a new base of aggregate and finished — along with the path — with a fine limestone gravel. It would be not only attractive and relatively easy to maintain — some weeding required — it would also be a permeable surface for stormwater runoff. It was an elegant, simple and cost-effective solution.

The project was winding down when, along with Superkül, we decided to engage a specialist in "green rating" to shepherd the LEED certification process. Since we had made a sincere effort to create a sustainably built, energy-efficient home within the overall context of a healthy house, we thought the minor additional cost was justified to have the certification at some level — probably Gold, with a fantasy of Platinum.

One note about LEED that you can learn from our experience: If you're interested in achieving certification for a new home, be sure to register your project before construction begins. Then hire an experienced green rater to ensure that all the LEED documentation is in order and the house is being built to the right specifications. It is much more complicated and time-consuming, or perhaps even impossible, to complete after the fact. The Canada Green Building Council attempts to make certification easy, but you should educate yourself about the process in advance. For an overview, see the Council's documentation on its requirements.[3,4]

New homes trying to qualify for LEED recognition are measured on a point system across eight major categories. As you can see from the number of points awarded in each category, the weight of the certification is on sustainability, energy efficiency, and indoor environmental quality:

- Innovation and Process Design (up to 11 points)

- Location and Linkages (10 points)

- Sustainable Sites (22 points)

- Water Efficiency (15 points)

- Energy and Atmosphere (38 points)

- Materials and Resources (16 points)

- Indoor Environmental Quality (21 points)

- Awareness and Education (3 points)

For a variety of reasons that had little to do with us or the house, the data gathering, rating analysis and final certification took years — too long and certainly not what the Canada Green Building Council has in mind for the homeowner's experience. But in the end, +*House* was awarded Gold certification by the LEED Canada for Homes rating system. As they said in their email to us announcing the award, "LEED Canada certification identifies your project as a pioneering example of sustainable design and demonstrates your leadership in transforming the building industry."

Notes

1   http://www.cagbc.org/cagbcdocs/CaGBC%20Media%20Kit.pdf

2   The email from the Envirolok rep, who was a great help to Jeff Pepper, stated: "Envirolok is the manufacturer and supplier of a green bioengineering methodology and system for building 3 dimensional mechanically interlocked soft vegetated earth-scaping systems for erosion control, retaining walls, slope stability & streambank protection. Envirolok has demonstrated appeal where immediate structural stability and integrity is required and a vegetated outcome is desired. Envirolok can be simply engineered to fit applications where conventional bioengineering or hard solutions can't work functionally or economically. Furthermore, with the inclusion of PermaMatrix, a Biotic Soil Amendment incorporating Biochar, Envirolok structures can sequester carbon for an added environmental benefit. "The Envirolok system employs a unique patented connector to provide 3-d interlocking strength to structures prior to vegetation, which can be accomplished by way of hydroseeding, live plugging, brush layering or live staking. The Envirolok system is an economical and environmentally friendly alternative to other soft bioengineering solutions and hardscaping materials such as gabion baskets, rip-rap, manufactured stone, armourstone or concrete."

3   http://www.cagbc.org/CAGBC/LEED/GreenHomes/Process/CAGBC/Programs/LEED/GreenHomes/The_Process.aspx?hkey=db106751-4342-47f6-bb13-b5afeb5d1b22

4   A more complete list of the CAGBC's supporting documents can be found at http://www.cagbc.org/CAGBC/LEED/GreenHomes/SupporDoc/CAGBC/Programs/LEED/GreenHomes/Supporting_Documents.aspx?hkey=84b37470-7d57-4f53-ba98-4c8b970b7219

Lesson 9:

Adding the "+" to Your House

Not everyone contemplating a healthier living environment will have the resources, inclination, or even the necessity of creating a prototype house like ours. Hiring and overseeing a small army of architects, contractors, sub-trades and suppliers, and engaging them in learning about healthy construction is a challenge to both your time and your finances. You will get an idea from the long list in the Appendix of the team who worked on *+House*.

Since you have come this far, let's assume that you're seriously considering creating a healthier living environment. The road you take will depend on your family's needs in a healthy home, especially the extent and type of environmental sensitivity that may already be affecting one or more of you. The appropriate approach will also depend on your financial and supervisory resources. The most important factor in the quality of the outcome, however, will be the depth of your interest in healthy building strategies, materials and processes.

As I hope is evident from the lessons in this book, ensuring that you're well informed about your own issues and construction options is the foundation not just for your intention to build healthy but also for your advocacy on behalf of yourself and your family. The status quo, for the most part, will be arrayed firmly against you. You must not let it overwhelm your goal for creating the healthiest living environment you can with the resources you have. The ideas and sources in this book, as well as the specific information to be found in the books and websites in the Appendix, are a good place to start your information-gathering.

What, then, are your options for a healthier house if you're not considering building a prototype for your geographic area and specific site? For example, what can you reasonably ask of a production builder putting up dozens of new homes in a subdivision? Are you thinking about building a custom house of relatively conventional construction? What strategies should you adopt if you have decided to renovate your existing home and want to ensure that it not only gives you the features you want but also the "clean" environment you need?

This chapter presents a handful of ideas that will help you navigate some of the important decisions you may wish to make in order to create the healthy, or at least healthier, home you seek. I am indebted to those who have contributed meaningfully to these ideas, especially John Godden, CEO of ClearSphere (**www.clearsphere.ca**) and a pioneering Canadian LEED consultant; Dr. Mark Cree Jackson, an expert on indoor environmental quality (**www.northamerica-daikin.com**); and the late Billy Ware, CEO of Ware Architectural Studios in Dallas (**www.warearchitecture.com**).

Basic Principles

Let's start with two deceptively simple but essential principles of healthy building that should be your touchstones for a great many decisions. They apply to both the construction materials used and to the electromagnetic (EMF) and radio-frequency (RF) radiation found in most conventionally built homes:

Principle 1: Don't put bad stuff in.
Principle 2: Filter out bad stuff that can't be avoided.

What do I mean, in very general terms, by Principle 1? Simply that you will get the best initial and ongoing indoor environmental quality if you don't use toxic materials in the first place. Think about the largest surfaces in the house, which will have the greatest impact on air quality — the floors, ceilings and walls. Floors, for example, play a major role depending on the quality — and method of installation — of the hardwood, tile, or carpet. Drywall quality, joint compounds, and paint used on the walls and ceiling can together be potent off-gassers. Glues and sealants, like those used in cabinetry manufacturing and kitchen countertop and window installation also add to the chemical stew that emanates from most conventional new construction. Included under this Principle are sources of electromagnetic (EMF) and radio frequency (RF) pollution from Wi-Fi, smart meters, cell phones and ill-considered or poorly installed electrical wiring. If possible, all of this "bad stuff" should be minimized or eliminated.

What about Principle 2 in general terms — filter out what you can't avoid? As builders have responded to evolving building codes and buyers seeking greater energy efficiency, houses have become more airtight. That traps pollutants in the house and eliminates the unintended ventilation that "leaky" houses once passively supplied. As a result, newer homes should be well ventilated with outside air. Unfortunately, outside air can itself introduce allergens like pollens, molds, pesticides, and automotive exhaust to the indoor mix. The solution to both issues is whole-house air filtration using a hierarchy of specialized equipment — depending on your needs and means — in conjunction with the forced-air distribution system. Again, this concept of filtration extends to EMF and RF pollution that is likely to be present in your new home or renovation. It's also worth noting that investing in active filtration will continue to deliver health benefits long after construction materials have off-gassed by cleaning the indoor air of "bad stuff" you produce just by living in the house — pet dander, dust mites, cooking smoke, excess humidity, and so on.

Lesson 6, *Look for the Unseen*, details many of the strategies we used in *+House* to align its construction, at least intuitively, with these principles. That's a good place to kick-start your thinking about what may be appropriate for your specific needs. I would also highly recommend consulting the books and websites listed in the Suggested Reading appendix. *Prescriptions for a Healthy House* in particular has very detailed chapters on the products, processes and rationale for achieving a healthier construction outcome. The book is organized by "divisions," which is how builders generally think about their projects, so if you're working with a contractor you may also want to insist they read *Prescriptions* as part of the contract.

Working with a Production Builder

For many people, often first-time buyers, a brand new house in a master-planned community provides the best opportunity for affordable home ownership. It's a smart decision in most ways. Production, or volume, builders who construct large numbers of houses every year offer generally well-built homes that are up to the latest building code requirements and come with strong warranty protections. Finishes can be customized to individual preferences. And these days, there are likely to be a host of built-in 'sustainability' features that will provide savings on energy costs and water usage.

That said, a production house is unlikely to offer the healthiest initial indoor air quality, and may not give you the tools you need for ongoing air quality even when most of the building materials have gassed off. So here's the question: If buying a home in a master-planned community is the right choice for your resources, and you need your new home to be as healthy as possible when you move in, what can you reasonably expect from your builder?

Unfortunately, not very much.

Earlier chapters detailed many of the issues we had with trades and suppliers for +*House* who didn't initially want to change their processes or materials to accommodate our quest to build healthy. That was a one-off custom home. A production builder in a subdivision may be constructing hundreds of homes based on a few standardized models, and they may have built thousands of similar houses over a period of years. They have proven processes in place that generate profits and ensure they can stand behind their warranties. They benefit from volume purchases of materials they can use across all units. Cabinetry is likely fabricated to precise specifications in a large, automated plant. Customization is generally limited to packages of finishes or relatively minor construction details that will add to the bottom line. We should not begrudge them running a profitable business, but these realities speak more to the builder's health than your own.

"The issue [of healthy building] is not well understood by the industry," I was told by one vice-president of construction for a major new-home builder in Ontario, who spoke off the record so he could be candid in his comments. "We have no real resource. We can't pull out the building code and look it up. We could Google the ideas but we wouldn't know if the practices were validated, and that's a problem for warranties."

It appears that builder responsiveness to healthy construction issues is driven primarily by legislation — the building code. In Ontario, for example, the code has stipulated a move away from solvent-based paints, glues, and laminates in recent revisions. Similarly, as homes have become more airtight and energy-efficient in recent years, requirements for improving indoor air quality have been written into the standards. The company

mentioned above was one of the first to voluntarily install heat-recovery ventilators (HRVs) in new homes to
bring in higher volumes of conditioned fresh air. Positive
changes like these are coming, but they do not seem to
be driven by consumers.

If you're considering purchasing a production home
in a hot real estate market, expect your salesperson to
be respectful of your health concerns but probably quite
inflexible in the package of upgrades they will want to
offer. Once you have chosen a building lot and house
design and secured them with your deposit, your time in
the builder's presentation center will probably be limited
to two or three visits, during which you will have the
opportunity to choose attractive packages of upgrades
to the basic house. That's enticing, but if you really have
a need for the best possible indoor environment in your
new home — "possible" meaning achievable and affordable — then you may want to consider a handful of
healthier options than spending the additional money
you have on standard builder upgrades. (If you can afford
both, great.) But here again, you may need to explain and
advocate for your health concerns either with the presentation center staff or with your assigned construction
manager. Be polite, but firm.

What, then, *can* you reasonably ask for from the
builder of your new house? Let's look at several important

options from the standpoint of our two principles. First, don't put bad stuff in in the first place:

Paint. Walls and ceilings represent the largest off-gassing surfaces in your home. Most reputable builders will be well aware of the argument for improved initial air quality and some will offer paint options that contain low or zero volatile organic compounds (VOCs). We have used zero VOC paints from AFM Safecoat and Sherwin-Williams' Harmony line. Both were excellent for our particular sensitivities as well as for application and durability. Another option to explore is mineral-based paints, which are manufactured from natural raw materials without petrochemical additives of any type. Mineral paints are available from Romabio (**http://romabio.com**) and Keim (**http://keim-usa.com**). Like zero-VOC paints, mineral coatings have a price tag of at least twice the cost of builder-grade paints, so expect to pay a premium if your builder agrees to use one of these alternatives. You will also need to order color chips and the paint you intend to use in advance, as these products are not typically available from home improvement warehouses.

Hardwood Floors. The possible combination of floor finishes in a new house is as varied as the number of new house designs. It's largely dependent on your builder, your home's price point and, ultimately, whatever upgrades you buy. In general, you will find a combination of hardwood, tile, and carpet. The ideal hardwood floor — and a more expensive option — will be made from solid hardwoods, prefinished at the factory and nailed to the subfloor; engineered hardwoods, in which pieces of wood are bound by glues, will off-gas for some time.

If the floor is to be finished onsite, try to stipulate a solvent- and formaldehyde-free stain such as AFM Safecoat DuroStain (**www.afmsafecoat.com**) and a protective coat of aluminum oxide rather than the more typically used polyurethane. If your builder will not budge on his way of doing things, before you move in consider treating the finished hardwood floors with AFM Safecoat Hard Seal, which forms a continuous membrane over the wood and effectively prevents it from off-gassing. (You may recall from Lesson 6 that this was our strategy for preventing off-gas from the cedar ceiling in *+House*.) Another alternative is to apply Vermeister Zero VOC Polyurethane Kit, which contains no volatile organic compounds, solvents or other toxic ingredients.

Carpet. Depending on your home's layout, the builder will likely specify wall-to-wall carpeting down the hallway (and possibly on the stairs) that lead to the bedrooms, as well as in the bedrooms themselves. As nice as wall-to-wall broadloom can feel underfoot, especially in cold climates, it is a poor choice for occupants with health concerns. Again, consider the large surface area of your floors. The carpet covering them will not just off-gas from its own products of manufacture and installation, it will also quickly become a gathering place for dust, dirt, bacteria, molds, pet dander, dust mites, and dirt tracked in from outside. Even with regular vacuuming it's almost impossible to consistently keep clean.

As an alternative to carpet, try to negotiate with your builder for solid hardwood stairs, or at least stair treads. A healthier option for hallways and bedrooms is naturally manufactured linoleum sheeting, or tiles like Marmoleum. Forbo Flooring Systems makes a wide range of very attractive products, which you will find at **www.forbo.com/flooring/en-gl/product-finder/ poczak#&application=RESID**. While it will off-gas to some degree, luxury vinyl flooring by manufacturers like Armstrong (**www.armstrong.com/flooring/prod-ucts/luxury-vinyl**) offers a wide variety of options and is readily available. Be sure to specify an adhesive like AFM Safecoat 3 in 1 Adhesive or Forbo Sustain 885 M Sheet and Tile Adhesive, a water-based, non-toxic prod-uct. In the absence of carpet, use throw rugs of either natural fibers or synthetics like viscose for comfort; rugs like these can be easily removed and cleaned.

Finally, it's quite possible your builder simply won't entertain the idea of an alternative floor covering. In that case, and if your budget will allow, ask for a high-quality wool option or one that is manufactured with completely synthetic materials, like viscose, or natural fibers such as sisal or seagrass. If possible, specify a broadloom that has not been treated with contaminants like moth-proofing, fire retardants, stain repellents, and antibacterials. A healthy approach to installation is also very important. Insist on a non-toxic underpadding using, for example, recycled fibers like felt. While laying carpet with tackless strips is always preferable to using glues, if glue is necessary, the Safecoat 3 in 1 Adhesive will be among the best options. Ask that the carpet seams be sealed with a low- or zero-VOC carpet tape. CHAPCO products are a good place to start your search (www.chapco-adhesive. com/green-building.cfm).

Last word: You should expect not only higher costs associated with process and product changes like these, but also the potential for limited warranties. Each of the products mentioned in these sections are proven performers but they may not be known to the builder and sub-trades — especially in terms of time to acquire, use, or install and their ability to stand up to normal use. Expect resistance!

In terms of our second principle and given some flexibility in your budget, what can you ask of a production builder to help filter out the bad stuff that may result from construction materials and processes? Let's look at some options you should consider pursuing.

Ventilation. Your first line of defense against the accumulated particulates and gases of new construction is to dilute their impact with abundant fresh air. Yes, you can open the windows, but that is often impractical in very hot or cold climates. Besides, open windows are a welcome mat for all manner of dust, pollens, molds, and other contaminants like exhaust fumes.

A whole-house ventilation solution for colder climates is the heat recovery ventilator (HRV). These units take the energy from outgoing indoor air to warm incoming fresh air, typically recovering about 70 percent of the energy already expended in heating. Energy recovery ventilators (ERV) are more appropriate for warmer climates, like the southern United States. ERVs remove humidity from incoming fresh air and transfer it to the stale indoor that is being exhausted to the outside of the house. In either case, insist on a unit with a variable speed fan and the capability, especially for the chemically sensitive, to completely change the air in the house at least once an hour on the highest setting. Expect to spend about $1,000 on this upgrade, plus installation. Note that very hot, cold or humid air may require additional equipment to get this rate of air turnover.

If you have another $1,200 to invest, consider requesting an upgrade to a direct-vent, sealed-combustion furnace with a DC (direct current) motor. This option will provide the furnace with combustion air from outside that will add to your home's air quality and do it at a much lower cost-to-operate than a conventional furnace.

Two other ventilation considerations. Since your stove is one of the largest single "polluters" in the home, make sure you have, and use, a large range hood that exhausts directly to the outside; this is a good place to consider an upgrade if one is available. And because excess moisture can be a precursor to mold issues, be sure to use the exhaust fan while showering. Consider a unit that shuts down only when the humidity in the bathroom has been reduced to less than 60 percent. Some HRVs and ERVs also come with a remote timer for bathroom areas that can increase the fan speed and air extraction for set periods of time. These will require additional wiring.

Air Filtration.[1] Even for healthy people, it makes good sense to get as many pollutants out of your new home as possible. New construction, your daily routines, and the outside environment result in a wide array of contaminants that can affect your home's indoor air quality and potentially your health. A good filtration system will effectively eliminate airborne particulates like dust, dust mites, smoke, and dander. It should remove what are known as "bio-aerosols" — living airborne particles such as bacteria, viruses, and fungi — as well as off-gases of VOCs from construction materials and furniture. Semi-volatile organic compounds (SVOCs) from the use of chemicals such as flame retardants, stain repellants, anti-microbial agents, and pesticides also need to be taken into consideration as they tend to adhere to dust particles as they break down and then accumulate inside the house. Ideally, compounds like these fall into under the "don't put bad stuff in" principle.[2]

As mentioned in Lesson 6, at *+House* we used the Lifebreath whole house system, (**http://www.lifebreath.com/products**) which comprises an HRV and an "upstream" turbulent flow precipitator that settles out large particulates. This protects the efficiency of the "downstream" HEPA ("high energy particulate air") filter — HEPA filters are prone to clogging if overloaded with particulate matter — and gives us "hospital grade," low-maintenance filtration. The installed cost for the Lifebreath model TFP3000HEPA system should be approximately $1,500.

The Lennox PureAir whole house system (**http://www.lennox.com/products/indoor-air-quality/air-purification/pureair**) is another high-quality product that effectively removes airborne particulates, bio-aerosols, and odors from the home. It combines "hospital quality," active charcoal air filtration with a germicidal ultra-violet light and a titanium dioxide metal mesh to filter odors. The installed cost for a PureAir system will be about $2,300; the filters and ultra-violet lamp must be replaced annually. Other major HVAC manufacturers such as Carrier, Daikin, and Trane also offer whole house filtration options.

Radon Rough-in. Radon is a naturally occurring, radioactive gas from decaying uranium found in soil and rock. Odorless, tasteless and invisible, it seeps into homes through cracks in the foundation, walls and joints and, depending on the concentration of the gas, presents a significant health threat to the occupants. According to the Environmental Protection Agency, radon is the second leading cause of lung cancer in the United States — and the leading cause of the disease among non-smokers. That's why it is highly recommended by both the EPA and Health Canada to regularly test your home for radon, ideally using a long-term test.[3]

What to do about getting rid of this naturally occurring but nevertheless bad stuff? More builders and building codes are specifying that new homes have a roughed-in system for venting radon to the outdoors should post-construction testing indicate levels above the minimum acceptable. This is a relatively simple, inexpensive procedure if done before the basement foundation or slab-on-grade is poured, but it is far more expensive if you must do it after the house is built. The contractor will lay a network of connected, perforated PVC pipe in the soil underneath the slab that allows the gases in the soil to collect. If tests show elevated levels of radon in the house, it is a simple matter to attach a small fan to the collector vent stack above grade to pull the accumulated radon out from under the foundation and into the outside air, where it will be harmless. The cost of this rough-in should range between $250 to $750 at the time of construction.

Central Vacuum System. While this feature may seem like an indulgence, it's really not if it's properly installed. For a family with health sensitivities, that means that the vacuum unit will exhaust particle-laden air directly to the outside of the home, not into, say, a closet in the garage.

Compare the cost of a central vac system to a high-quality conventional vacuum cleaner with a HEPA filter such as a Miele, which is discussed below. Central vacs are also built-in appliances that can add to the overall value of your home. If you go this route, be sure to empty the vacuum canister and change filters regularly.

Electrical Fields. You may recall that my wife, Barbara, experienced feelings of "spikiness" while inspecting a house we were considering buying. For some people, that kind of hypersensitivity to electrical fields is their constant condition, leading to debilitating symptoms such as insomnia, depression and anxiety. Prolonged sleeplessness is often a side-effect of this sensitivity.

You can reduce electric fields by asking your builder's electrical contractor to install a kill switch that will cut off power to an individual circuit. The bedroom, or bedrooms, are a good place to start because electricity is usually not needed during sleeping hours and your body needs that time to regenerate free of aggravating electrical fields. Simply turn off the switch before climbing into bed to cut power to the circuit.

You or your home's construction manager will need to work with the electrician to plan the most effective placement of kill switches. Obviously, power should not be cut off to essential appliances like smoke detectors, carbon monoxide alarms and the refrigerator. But because there are numerous important technical considerations to be taken into account, I suggest you first consult the section on kill and demand switches in *Prescriptions for a Healthy Home* and insist the electrician read those sections prior to making modifications to the wiring plan.

Connectivity. The construction executive mentioned earlier noted during our conversation that their new homes offer Ethernet connections in every room. "It doesn't get used," he said. "Customers always ask for more Wi-Fi, never less of it." That's fine, unless someone in your family is sufficiently sensitive to radio frequencies that Wi-Fi exacerbates their symptoms. Then you must turn off the Wi-Fi and plug in your computers. Consider an upgrade from the typical Cat 5 wiring to Cat 6, which boosts maximum network throughput speed from one to 10 gigabits per second up to a maximum of 150 feet from the internet router. That's certainly more through-put than any individual needs for current technologies, but it is one area where you can easily "future proof" your new home, and add to its resale value, by enabling the addition of wired smart hubs and other to-be-developed conveniences—if not for you, for the next owner.

Less-Costly Options

If you can convince your builder to make the changes that are most important for your family, and you can afford them, that's great. But what can you do to protect your health if your builder is unwilling to make the changes you've requested, or you just can't afford the additional costs of alternative materials and whole-house air filtration? Here are a few ideas with relatively low price tags:

Passive Ventilation. Open the windows to accelerate the turnover of stale air, especially during the first few months after construction when materials are off-gassing. If you take possession of your new home during winter in a cold climate, this may limit you to a few minutes at a time, but it is worth the short-term discomfort (and slightly higher heating costs) to get toxic off-gases out. Consider opening all cabinet doors at night for a few months so they can off-gas more quickly and be diluted and ventilated out with the air turnover.

Furnace Filters. Minimum Efficiency Reporting Value (MERV) is an industry standard that rates the overall effectiveness of the air filters that are part of your home's heating, ventilation and air-conditioning (HVAC) system. MERV ratings range from 1 to 16; the higher the rating the finer the filtration, meaning fewer dust particles and other airborne pollutants can pass through the filter. Your builder has likely installed a basic one-inch pleated filter with an adequate rating, say a MERV 6. This will remove up to 50 percent of particles from 3-10 microns — pollen, dust, dust mites and most mold spores. (For comparison, a human hair is about 100 microns wide.)

For better air quality, consider using one-inch MERV 11 filters such as 3M's Filtrete Ultra Allergen 1500 (Purple). These will remove more than 85 percent of particles 3-10 microns as well as up to 80 percent of those from 1-3 microns in size. In addition to removing larger particles, these filters will also remove smoke, smog, bacteria, and virus-carrying particles from your home. The MERV 13 Filtrete Elite Allergen 2200 will remove progressively more particulates as well as particles that carry odors.[4] Consider changing the filters monthly for the first six months after construction, then every three months thereafter. Filtrete filters are widely available at home improvement warehouses and online suppliers in a price range of $18 to $25 each. Well worth it.

When you can afford it, explore the benefits of installing a four-to-five-inch MERV 13 particulate filter or an active carbon filtration system. While some modification to your HVAC system will be necessary to accommodate these wider filters, they remove all of the particulates noted above as well as off-gases from volatile organic compounds. Filters should be changed annually.

Vacuum Cleaner. As effective as your furnace air filters may be, they remove primarily airborne particulates. Heavier particles like those from dust, pollen, dust mites, pet dander, and semi-volatile organic compounds will typically fall quickly to surfaces like floors, carpets, furniture and cabinetry and are no longer airborne unless your daily activities dislodge them. That's actually an opportunity for healthier indoor air quality rather than a problem needing to be cleaned up — if you approach the clean-up correctly.

Most vacuum cleaners don't do a very good job of filtering the air that exhausts from the unit. That can result in a room that actually has more airborne particulates after cleaning than before. Look for a good-quality unit with a HEPA filter, which should remove more than 99 percent of all particulates and allergens. Vacuum all surface areas — carpeting, rugs, hardwood, tile, furniture — at least weekly and more often if you have pets. And be sure to change or clean the filters regularly, preferably outside your living space.

Re-clean. It's almost certain that your builder will have done a comprehensive post-construction cleaning before handing over the keys to your new home. Your need for and definition of clean may be quite different, however. I suggest a thorough re-clean of the entire house, especially the tops and insides of cabinetry and drawers. Damp-wipe surfaces and vacuum if needed. Pay attention to the tops of window and door frames and any residue on window sills that could blow in when the windows are opened. And don't forget closets and storage spaces: anywhere that tends to be closed up will take longer to off-gas from paints, caulking, carpeting, and other chemicals.

If you and your family are sensitive to the chemicals in cleaning products, or want to ensure you make a healthier choice, please see the list of products we use at *+House* in Lesson 7. For a more comprehensive and objective listing, check out the Environmental Working Group's evaluation of 2,500 household cleaning products at **http://www.ewg.org/guides/cleaners**.

Smart Meter. As noted in Lesson 6, "Living in the Field," and in the endnotes, the controversy about the effects of smart meter radio radiation on neurological well-being continues to rage. Personally, we believe that a device which pulses radio signals thousands of times an hour and has a communication range of five miles or more should be cause for concern. If you feel that reducing pulsed radiation from your smart meter is necessary, consider installing a smart meter guard. This easily-installed product uses Faraday cage technology to block up to 99 percent of the radiation emitted by the meter, without compromising the data it sends back to the utility company. See **http://smartmeterguard.com**. Expect to pay $130 to $150, depending on currency.

Wi-Fi. There is no question that Wi-Fi signals, like cell signals, are ubiquitous these days. Like the health effects of smart meters, the impact of Wi-Fi signals on the brain, heart, and cells remains a very contentious issue among researchers. The test of whether or not to have Wi-Fi in your home should be yours. If you feel more relaxed and focused without it — assuming you have tried to live without it — use your Ethernet connection instead. If you decide it's fine, it makes sense to place the Wi-Fi router away from the bedroom areas so the signals don't contribute to the potential for sleep disruptions. Another good strategy is to turn off the Wi-Fi radio using the router's software before you go to bed, then turn it back on again in the morning, a simple process. The only cost is a few seconds of your time. Note that you will need a wired connection to the router to be able to turn the Wi-Fi back on.

Bigger Projects

At the beginning of this chapter, I asked whether you are considering building a custom house of relatively conventional construction or if you have decided to renovate your existing home and want to ensure that it gives you not only the features you want but also the "clean" environment you need.

While many of the ideas and materials highlighted throughout this book are readily applicable to both major renovations and custom construction, it is well beyond my level of understanding to make recommendations for complex projects. There are simply too many products and processes for the layperson to take into account, let alone their implications for creating a healthy built environment. That task is best left to the experts. Fortunately, there are a growing number of those. Here are links to a few resources that can get you to the expertise you will need:

The **U.S. Green Building Council**, which oversees LEED certification and education programs, offers a service called Green Home Guide (**http://www.greenhomeguide.com**) that enables you to search their database of 17,000 green building professionals worldwide, though mostly in the United States.

Like its U.S. counterpart, the **Canada Green Building Council** is focused on advocacy, education, and certification and so provides portals to experts in green construction and renovation on its LEED for Homes pages. You will find registered companies that can help with new construction at **https://www.cagbc.org/CAGBC/Programs/ LEED/GreenHomes/LEEDforHomeowners/ Building_a_green_hom.aspx** .

For renovation projects, see **https://www.cagbc. org/CAGBC/Programs/LEED/GreenHomes/ LEEDforHomeowners/Expert_Resources_for.aspx**.

Unfortunately, at present both are short lists.

Although better indoor air quality is an important measure in LEED for Homes certification, it may not be good enough for your family's health issues. Moreover, LEED does not take into account issues of electromagnetic and radio frequency pollution.

If "green" and "clean" don't necessarily align in terms of your needs, consider seeking out a Certified Building Biologist. The **International Institute for Building-Biology® and Ecology** (IBE) is a nonprofit educational organization based in Santa Fe, New Mexico. Building biologists accredited through IBE are trained in proven methods for ensuring that virtually any built space is as free as possible from indoor toxins and electromagnetic pollution — see the 25 Principles of Building Biology in the Appendix. They can be great accomplices in realizing your intention to build a healthier home. Recall that in Lesson 4 I described our meeting with Robert Stellar, a deeply experienced building biologist in Ontario and former IBE board member. It was an encounter that meaningfully enhanced the healthy qualities in our home. You can find a listing of Certified Building Biologists on IBE's website at **http://hbelc.org**.

Whether you're doing a renovation or a new build, you will find that the process of selecting your construction team will demand that you be the clearest and most vocal advocate for the healthiest living environment you can create. But while you may be clear in your individual intention, there is no substitute for a common intention with your contractor, and the contractor with his subtrades. A shared belief in what is possible is essential not only to get through the challenges of healthy building but also to the creation of a sanctuary of healing and regeneration for you and your family. That's the most satisfying lesson we learned in creating +*House*.

Notes

1   For an extensive discussion of the types of pollutants air cleaners remove, the performance of various types of air cleaners and the reduction of adverse health effects you can expect, see this study by the U.S. Environmental Protection Agency: **https://www.epa.gov/indoor-air-quality-iaq/guide-air-cleaners-home#will-air-cleaning-reduce**

2   You will find a useful academic overview of SVOCs (Table 1 is especially informative) at **http://surface.syr.edu/cgi/viewcontent.cgi?article=1009&context=mae**.

3   Health Canada offers a good overview of the need for regular testing and testing procedures at **http://healthycanadians.gc.ca/security-securite/radiation/radon/home-test-maison-eng.php**

4   You will find a handy comparison chart of these filters at **http://www.iallergy.com/filtrete-air-filter-comparison.php**.

Epilogue

The success of any home construction, conventional or healthy, is ultimately in the living. How does the built space support whatever intention you hold for your new dwelling?

Our mandate for *+House* was to create a sanctuary that would support Barbara's healing and well-being while we were there. (Mine, too, of course.) To accomplish that, we needed the house to be free of stressors like off-gassing materials and electromagnetic frequencies that typically pollute modern homes. As this book details, we achieved our mandate, and then some. We feel there is a tangible 'softness' to the living space that derives from the abundance of light, the clay wall finishes, and the serenity of the views. Equally relaxing are the elegant, uncluttered lines of the design and the neutral palette of the finishes and furniture. More prosaically, but equally important, its combination of size, design, and materials enables us to easily maintain the cleanliness we need for health and comfort. So, after five years of living in *+House,* it continues to delight us, and those who visit, in every way.

Our team's success in finding a balance of good design and healthy design has been echoed in awards *+House* has received since it was completed. I include them here not as a pat on our own backs as clients but as an acknowledgement of trailblazing work done by the architects, contractor, and trades to bring the original idea into reality.

In May 2012, for example, Superkül was honored with a coveted Award of Excellence from the Ontario Association of Architects, which judged *+House* on its creativity, sustainability, and response to its context. The house won a Residential Wood Design Award in the 2012 Wood WORKS! Ontario Awards, a project of the Canadian Wood Council. And in the fall of 2013, the house was named a winner of a Best of Canada Design Award by *Canadian Interiors* magazine. Numerous Canadian publications and international architecture blogs have also featured the house and its construction. But no acknowledgement said it better — at least to those of us who lived through its evolution from concept to realization — than the contemporary architecture and design magazine *Azure,* which stated in its May 2012 edition that +*House* set "... a new precedent in Canadian environmental design."

The leading edge of any big change, like that of healthy building, can be a lonely place for advocates. Unless prompted by need, few people are aware of, or even particularly interested in, the advantages that a healthy home can bestow. Fewer still will have an absolute need like ours to create a safe living space. Public awareness is slow to embrace materials and processes that would be good for anyone, especially when there may be added costs for healthier options. Some building codes are now mandating improved indoor air quality through better ventilation systems. And the availability (and affordability) of products like paints, adhesives, insulation, flooring, and so on that do not off-gas has expanded considerably since Superkül developed the original specifications for +*House* in 2010.

Nevertheless, we've watched with a bit of disappointment as siblings, cousins, and friends — with only a couple of exceptions — undertook new construction or major renovations without asking us a single question about our well-publicized experience and what we might recommend to avoid or at least reduce the effects of the building materials they were using. Superkül and Wilson Project Management do question clients about sensitivities to construction materials, but neither of them is regularly asked to specifically create a healthy living or working environment. The lack of demand for better options shouldn't be surprising, yet it is — at least to our evangelical instincts.

The inertia that limits public awareness of healthy building alternatives underscores the importance of two broad imperatives in this book. First, you must know yourself and your health situation with as much clarity as you can muster. And, second, you must be a vocal advocate for a creating a living environment that will support your healing. Barbara, to her great credit, was unwavering on both counts. I can attest that her "dark night" stretched out to what became dark years. But it was the strength of her resolve to get better — aided by many fine professional resources — that ultimately helped her gain momentum on her healing journey. +*House* was just one step along the way, but a step whose importance cannot be overstated.

Acknowledgments

With gratitude for the original inspiration for this book to Amedeo Barbini, custom builder extraordinaire, and to Garry Lester, who encouraged me to pursue my own voice. To John Godden, Dr. Mark Cree Jackson, and the late Billy Ware for sharing their deep professional knowledge of healthy living environments. To André D'Elia, Geoffrey Moote, Andy Johnson, Jeff Pepper, and Tim Singbeil for their willingness to submit to my interview questions. To Barbara Eastman, Rick Margerison, Marianne McKenna, and Fred Shoemaker whose insights and encouragement helped me get across the finish line. To editor Douglas Williams, who brought clarity to the manuscript. And to my wife, Barbara, whose healing journey prompted this one. The grace and fortitude with which you face the daily challenges of living healthy are an inspiration to all who know you.

Appendix

In addition to references in the various endnotes throughout the book, the following are a few of the resources that we have found useful in building and maintaining +*House*:

Suggested Reading

Baker-Laporte, Paula, Elliott, Erica, Banta, John, *Prescriptions for a Healthy House: A Practical Guide for Architects, Builders and Homeowners*, Third Edition. New Society Publishers, 2008.

Berman, Alan, *Green Design: A Healthy Home Handbook*, Revised Edition. Frances Lincoln Limited Publishers, 2008.

Environmental Protection Agency, *Indoor Air Quality: An Introduction for Health Professionals*. 2016. Available at **https://www.epa.gov/indoor-air-quality-iaq/indoor-air-pollution-introduction-health-professionals**

Gorman, Carolyn, *Less-Toxic Alternatives*, Tenth Edition. Optimum Publishing, 2010.

Hobbs, Angela, *The Sick House Survival Guide: Simple Steps to Healthier Homes*. New Society Publishers, 2003.

Jenkins, McKay, *What's Gotten into Us? Staying Healthy in a Toxic World*, Random House, 2011.

Rapp, Doris J., M.D., *Our Toxic World: A Wake-Up Call*, Environmental Medical Research Foundation, 2004

Rea, William J., M.D., *Optimum Environments for Optimum Health & Creativity Designing and Building a Healthy Home or Office*. Crown Press, Inc., 2002.

Smith, Rick and Lourie, Bruce, *Slow Death by Rubber Duck: The Secret Danger of Everyday Things*. Counterpoint Press, Kindle Edition, 2011.

Thompson, Athena, *Homes that Heal*. New Society Publishers, 2004.

Useful Websites

The **Agency for Toxic Substances and Disease Registry** (ATSDR) is a federal public health agency of the U.S. Department of Health and Human Services. ATSDR provides health information to prevent harmful exposures and diseases related to toxic substances. **https://www.atsdr.cdc.gov**

With a mission to protect human health and the environment, the United States **Environmental Protection Agency** provides a very deep resource of information on health and building issues. **https://www.epa.gov**

EcoHome is an excellent site on sustainable building techniques and materials for builders and homeowners. **http://www.ecohome.net**

The **Environmental Working Group** is a research and education organization dedicated to "empowering people to live healthier lives in a healthier environment." **http://www.ewg.org**

Health Canada's goal is to help Canadians maintain and improve their health through research, consultation, and communication. Like the EPA site, Health Canada

offers useful information of great depth and breadth.
http://www.hc-sc.gc.ca/index-eng.php

The **Healthy Building Network** focuses on the role of
building materials in advancing environmental, health,
and social outcomes. While primarily focused on commercial construction, HBN is a leading voice in bringing
transparency to the composition and health impact of
building materials. **https://healthybuilding.net**

The Healthy Building Network's **Pharos Project** is one
of the most comprehensive (and independent) databases
for identifying health hazards associated with building
products. Now it its third iteration, the database cata-
logues 1,600 building products from more than 300
manufacturers, and profiles 37,500 chemicals and materials for health and environmental hazards. **https://
www.healthybuilding.net/content/pharos-v3**

The **International Institute for Building-Biology® and
Ecology** offers courses, seminars, and certifications in
creating healthy living environments. A good resource
for finding accredited Building Biologists in your area.
http://hbelc.org

The 25 Principles of Building Biology

Building materials and noise control

1. Use natural and unadulterated building materials.

2. A building shall have a pleasant or neutral smell, not releasing any toxins.

3. Use building materials with the lowest possible level of radioactivity.

4. Protective measures against noise and vibration pollution need to be based on human needs.

Indoor climate

5. Regulate indoor air humidity naturally by using humidity-buffering materials.

6. The total moisture content of a new building shall be low and dry out quickly.

7. Strive for a well-balanced ratio between thermal insulation and heat retention.

8. Optimize indoor surface and air temperatures of a given space.

9. Promote good indoor air quality through natural ventilation.

10. Use radiant heat for heating.

11. Interfere as little as possible with the natural balance of nature's own background radiation.

12. Prevent exposures to human-made sources of electromagnetic fields and radio-frequency radiation.

13. Minimize exposures to mold, bacteria, dust, and allergens.

The environment, energy, and water

14. Minimize energy consumption while using renewable energy whenever possible.

15. Prefer regional building materials, not promoting the exploitation of scarce and hazardous resources.

16. Building activities shall cause no environmental problems.

17. Choose the best possible drinking water quality.

Interior design

18. Take harmonic measures, proportions, and shapes into consideration.

19. Select light exposures, lighting systems, and color schemes following natural conditions.

20. Base interior and furniture design on physiological and ergonomic findings.

Building site

21. Site buildings on land free from geological and human-made disturbances.

22. Locate residential homes away from pollutant and noise sources.

23. Provide low-density housing with sufficient green space.

24. Develop individualized housing and settlements in harmony with nature in ways that support human and family needs.

25. Building activities shall cause no social problems.

© *Institut fur Baubiologie + Nachhaltigkeit IBN*

The +*House* Team

Architects

Superkül Inc., Toronto

Lead architect: André D'Elia, BArch, OAA, MRAIC

Project architect: Geoffrey Moote, MArch, LEED AP

Consulting Architect

Marianne McKenna, OC, MArch, OAA, OAQ, FRAIC, AIA

Project Management

Wilson Project Management, Collingwood, Ontario

Site Supervisor: Jeff Pepper

Accounting: Wendy Sholtz

Electrical & Mechanical Engineers

Rice Kong Engineering Limited, Toronto

Geotechnical Engineers

Terraprobe Inc., Brampton, Ontario

Consulting Engineer (Soil)

Richardson Foster Ltd., Barrie, Ontario

Structural Engineers

Blackwell Bowick Partnership Limited, Toronto

Insurance

Trillium Mutual Insurance, Listowel, Ontario

Noble Insurance, Collingwood, Ontario (agent)

Major Trades & Suppliers

Appliances

Macdonald's Furniture & Appliances, Meaford, Ontario

Concrete Floor

Rowland Concrete Services Limited, Tottenham, Ontario

Lafarge North America (concrete)

Demolition, Excavation, Haulage

Brian Dinsmore Excavation & Haulage Limited, Thornbury, Ontario

Electrical Contractor

Tri-Unite Systems Ltd., Toronto, Ontario

Electrical Supply

Torbram Electrical Supply, Toronto, Ontario

Eurolite, Toronto, Ontario

Fiberglass Rebar & Durisol Block

Durisol Building Systems Inc., Burlington, Ontario
Fiberglass Rebar & Durisol Block Installation, Parging
Dasein Homes Incorporated, Owen Sound, Ontario

Footings & Retaining Wall

Grey-Bruce Construction Limited, Mildmay, Ontario

Foundation Waterproofing

Advanced Coatings Inc., Midland, Ontario

Framing, Interior & Exterior Carpentry

Jorgenson Construction, Collingwood, Ontario
Darren McFarland, Collingwood, Ontario

Furniture

Italinteriors, Toronto, Ontario
Kiosk Design Inc., Toronto, Ontario

Green Roof System

Xeroflor Canada Inc., Toronto, Ontario

Hydronic Heating (Pond-Loop Geothermal)

B & R Hearth and Geothermal, Nottawa, Ontario

Insulation

Great Northern Insulation, Woodstock, Ontario

Interior Doors & Frames, Trim

Brenlo Ltd., Toronto, Ontario

Irrigation, Landscape Lighting & Hydroseeding

Georgian Sprinklers, Stayner, Ontario

Organic Express, Paris, Ontario

Landscaping

Zeng Landscaping, Creemore, Ontario

Sherri Wilson, Creemore, Ontario

Envirolok Canada, Kitchener, Ontario

Kitchen & Bathroom Glass

Barrie Metro Glass Inc., Barrie, Ontario

Millwork

Andrew Johnston Woodworking, Toronto, Ontario

Plumbing

Baymount Plumbing Ltd., Collingwood, Ontario (rough-in, install)

McKeough Supply Inc., Collingwood, Ontario (fixtures)

Roof & Skylights

Sky High Roofing & Renovations Inc., Barrie, Ontario

Septic System

Brian Dinsmore Excavation & Haulage Limited, Thornbury, Ontario

Premier Tech Acqua (Ecoflo Septic System)

Structural Steel

Thornbury Steel Fabricators Ltd., Thornbury, Ontario

Surveyors

Martin W. Knisley, OLS, Duntroon, Ontario

Zubek Emo Patten & Thomsen Limited, Collingwood, Ontario (foundations)

Tile Installation

Quanbury Flooring Centre, Stayner, Ontario

Wall Finishing

JW Custom Finish Inc., Pontypool, Ontario

Water System

Bosco Home Services, Mississauga, Ontario (Ecowater treatment system)

Culligan Canada, Orangeville, Ontario (kitchen reverse osmosis system)

Well Drilling
Jim Clarke Well Drilling Ltd., Meaford, Ontario

Windows
Radiant City Millwork Inc., Toronto, Ontario

Window Coverings
Brading Specialty Shades, Toronto, Ontario
Solarfective Products Ltd., Scarborough, Ontario

Other Suppliers
ADT Canada
Astley-Gilbert Limited (printing)
Annette Shaw
Bear Canyon Cabinet Company Ltd.
Bill Brown Woodworking & Builders Supply
Brad Rice (general labor)
CRS Contractors Rental Supply
Crystal Tile & Marble Ltd.
Dan Sinclair (tree care)
Design Within Reach
Eco Inhabit
Empire Hardware Limited
Eurolite
Federal Express

Flesherton Concrete Products
Hamilton Bros. Building Supplies
Havens Home Building Centre
Hill 'n Dale Landscaping
Hockley Rural High-Speed Internet
Huronia Recycling Limited
Jay D. Morgan
James T. Hill Painting
John Noble Septic
Miele Limited
Mountain Moving & Storage
Pro-Seal Caulking
Red Brick Group (entertainment center)
Robinson's Paint & Wallpaper Ltd.
Rona Ontario
Samuel Plate Sales (steel plate)
Staples
Stayner Rental
The Home Depot
The Zero Point
Tim-Br Mart
Torbram Electrical Supply
Total Electrical Supply Limited
Van Wyck Crane Service
Wayne Bird Fuels
Wildflower Farm

Appendix